Back to Life,
Back to Normality
Volume 2

Back to Life, Back to Normality Volume 2

CBT Informed Recovery for Families with Relatives with Schizophrenia and Other Psychoses

Edited by

Douglas Turkington
Northumberland, Tyne & Wear NHS Foundation Trust
Newcastle University

Helen M. Spencer
Northumberland, Tyne & Wear NHS Foundation Trust
Newcastle University

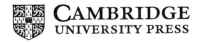
CAMBRIDGE
UNIVERSITY PRESS

CAMBRIDGE
UNIVERSITY PRESS

University Printing House, Cambridge CB2 8BS, United Kingdom

One Liberty Plaza, 20th Floor, New York, NY 10006, USA

477 Williamstown Road, Port Melbourne, VIC 3207, Australia

314–321, 3rd Floor, Plot 3, Splendor Forum, Jasola District Centre, New Delhi – 110025, India

79 Anson Road, #06-04/06, Singapore 079906

Cambridge University Press is part of the University of Cambridge.

It furthers the University's mission by disseminating knowledge in the pursuit of education, learning, and research at the highest international levels of excellence.

www.cambridge.org
Information on this title: www.cambridge.org/9781107564831
DOI: 10.1017/9781316410523

First published 2019

Printed and bound in Great Britain by Clays Ltd, Elcograf S.p.A.

A catalogue record for this publication is available from the British Library.

ISBN 978-1-107-56483-1 Paperback

Contents

Endorsements

At the Schizophrenia Society of Ontario we recognise and understand the challenges many caregivers experience when trying to care for and support a family member living with schizophrenia.

Caregivers are motivated and want to do their best but often don't know how and don't have the resources they need. Many caregivers have shared their feelings of being overwhelmed, helpless and hopeless.

Through our partnership and work with Dr Turkington, we were able to collaborate on a new and exciting initiative for caregivers, which has culminated in the creation of a one-of-a-kind, practical skill building programme, Cognitive Behaviour Therapy for Psychosis (CBTp): Informed Training for Caregivers.

In the spring and fall of 2016, CBTp: Informed Caring for Caregivers training was delivered in Ontario, Canada, which we facilitated alongside Dr Douglas Turkington. The caregiver training, offered through a two-day introductory-level workshop and a five-day intensive workshop, provides family members with new skills and tools which can improve caregiver support and resilience and enhance communication between the caregiver and their family member.

The feedback we received from caregivers tells us that we have successfully addressed a critical need. Caregivers told us that the training taught them practical skills and tools which they could now apply to their own circumstances and goals. This newfound knowledge has helped them to have more empathy for their family member and listen more effectively, and has helped caregivers make sense of their family member's experiences. Caregivers also told us that they experienced a sense of empowerment and hope for the future at the end of this training.

We are delighted with our collaboration with Dr Turkington and believe the impact of this initiative has been life changing for caregivers.

Mary Alberti, CEO
Schizophrenia Society of Ontario

Testimonials

'Since the program I have used the techniques with my family member. It's easier now to recognize their triggers, and understand their beliefs and thoughts. There is still a lot of information for me to go over but I believe that my family member can get better and live well'.

'Listening to my son was worthwhile, with no judgement, no advice, no ridicule. He told me later, when he was well, that he was aware that I was listening to him, and that it was very helpful to him. Now that he is doing better, I suggest ways to test his reasoning if it seems off. He is often able to see the logic'.

'In the past a professional had to encourage our family to learn how to 'talk' with our family member but our family lacked the skills and knowledge on how to do this – never knew what it was. CBTp training provided an opportunity to see from a different perspective and changed my way of thinking'.

'Recently my son was experiencing a lot of anxiety – in the past I would not have known what to say or how to support him ... I felt helpless. Through my CBTp training [I] was able to apply some of the communication techniques I learned and retained from my training and was able to communicate with him in a supportive manner. Later my son turned to me and said, "Thanks Mom – I feel a lot better." I felt so empowered and positive'.

'The training helped me to develop my own awareness and confidence building of awareness of "what to do and say" and "what not to do"'.

'Prior to taking the CBTp training I was unable to cope much longer with my family member, was exhausted and ready to run away. I registered for the two-day training which I found to be "really amazing" and was so taken and energized by the training I registered at the last minute for the five-day training. Since taking the training and applying some of what I learned my son has begun to open up to me. I am now committed to building on my CBT knowledge. My son recently said, "Mom there's no point in talking to you because you never listen" to which I stopped and replied "you're right – I haven't been listening" – remembering and applying some of the techniques I learned in the training – use short responses and learn to listen. My son then opened up and began talking!'

'Personally it provided me with hope in general and hope of effective treatment for people who were not doing well just taking meds alone – needed talk therapy for trauma'.

'Fabulous front line training for family members! Loved the role playing, small group size of the five-day training, interacting with others attending, networking, listening to and learning from other people's experiences, learning and becoming more knowledgeable on CBT'.

'Following the training I decided CBT could most definitely help my loved one and I was able to locate a CBT professional in private practice for my loved one. My loved one is now receiving CBT weekly and is very engaged in her treatment and sessions. I have new found hope'.

'Hope, Recovery, Befriending, and Normalizing is what I took away from Dr Turkington's two and five day intense hands on training about Cognitive Behaviour Therapy for Psychosis (CBTp) for caregivers. The CBTp training gave me the understanding of my son's illness with Schizophrenia and I became more **Confident** within myself. My son and I have a strong relationship now and he trusts me! CBTp informed training for caregivers is such a **Life Changing** program and [I] believe so strongly in [it], that I am now a volunteer with the Schizophrenia Society of Ontario (SSO) to advocate for Dr. Turkington's Informed CBTp training for carers and to help others'.

Contributors

Matt Brown, PhD
University of Texas Health Science Center at San Antonio, Texas, USA.

Suzanne Bell, PhD
Royal Ottawa Mental Health Centre, Ottawa, Canada.

Rea Cheetham, DClinPsy
Northumberland
Tyne and Wear NHS Foundation Trust, UK.

Thomas Christodoulides, DClinPsy
Northumberland
Tyne and Wear NHS Foundation Trust, UK.

Daniel Collerton, MSc
Northumberland
Tyne and Wear NHS Foundation Trust, UK and Newcastle University, UK.

David Couper
No affiliation (based in Newcastle upon Tyne, UK).

Maggie Douglas-Bailey, MSc
Northumberland
Tyne and Wear NHS Foundation Trust, UK

Robert Dudley, PhD
Northumberland
Tyne and Wear NHS Foundation Trust, UK and Newcastle University, UK.

Katherine Elliott, PhD
Tertiary Mental Health Services, Hospitals and Community Integrated Services, Kamloops, British Columbia, Canada.

Paul Gilbert, PhD, OBE
Centre for Compassion Research and Training, University of Derby, UK.

Charles Heriot-Maitland, DClinPsy
University of Glasgow, UK.

Latoyah Lebert, BSc
Northumberland
Tyne and Wear NHS Foundation Trust, UK and Newcastle University, UK

Eleanor Longden, PhD
Greater Manchester Mental Health NHS Foundation Trust, UK.

David Kingdon, MD
Southampton University, UK and Southern Health NHS Foundation Trust.

Jeremy Pelton, RMN
The Insight-CBT Partnership, UK.

Robert Reiser, PhD
University of California, San Francisco, USA.

Nazneen Rustom, BA
Carleton University, Ottawa, Canada.

Samuel Sargeant, MA
Cardiff University, UK.

Helen M. Spencer
Northumberland,
Tyne and Wear NHS Foundation Trust, UK and Newcastle University, UK.

Lucy Helen Stevens, DClinPsy
Tees, Esk and Wear Valleys NHS Foundation Trust, UK.

Douglas Turkington
Northumberland,
Tyne and Wear NHS Foundation Trust, UK and Newcastle University, UK.

Dawn Irene Velligan, PhD
University of Texas Health Science Center
at San Antonio, Texas, USA.

Nicola Patricia Wright, PhD
The Royal Ottawa Mental Health Centre,
Ottawa, Canada.

Foreword

Cognitive therapy principles and techniques are being increasingly applied beyond the arena of expert therapy. Correcting distorted thought processes and modifying our unrealistic beliefs about the self and others are important approaches which can be deployed across the span of human interaction. They can be applied within a marriage, in the boardroom or within a complex international negotiation. This volume examines how cognitive therapy approaches can be used by family members and caregivers of those with persistent psychotic symptoms and poor social functioning. Caregivers and those in close contact with individuals suffering from psychosis are optimally placed to catalyse recovery as they spend much more time in the company of their loved one than any mental health professional. Additionally, the volume aims to help caregivers use cognitive approaches to improve their own emotional health and balance their activities.

This book realistically and empathetically discusses the experience of psychosis and broadens the reader's understanding of the nature and persistence of psychotic symptoms. The authors focus on the importance of communication and indicate the optimal styles when interacting with individuals diagnosed with schizophrenia. Detailed information is given regarding how to care for a relative with paranoia, as well as effective coping strategies. Finally, novel areas such as how to help with visions and traumatic experiences are explored.

The result is a book which will be welcomed by caregivers, friends and family members. It will also serve as a tool for students learning cognitive therapy for schizophrenia and other forms of psychoses. I am happy to warmly endorse and recommend this book for professionals and consumers alike.

Aaron T. Beck, M.D.
Professor Emeritus of Psychiatry,
Department of Psychiatry,
University of Pennsylvania,
Philadelphia, PA, USA

Preface

This volume follows on from our previous book *Back to Life: Back to Normality: Cognitive Therapy, Recovery and Psychosis* which was published in 2009 by Cambridge University Press. The book was written for carers of those with schizophrenia, for those suffering with psychosis and as a primer for interested mental health professionals. The book was well received and the present volume further develops the concept of CBT informed caring as a safe and viable catalyst for recovery. Carers and friends spend more time with the person with schizophrenia than psychiatrists, psychologists, psychiatric nurses, social workers or occupational therapists. As such they are in a unique position to help deliver a carefully constructed treatment plan. We know that the prognosis is good in 60 per cent of people who develop a first episode of schizophrenia. At long-term follow-up over 20–30 years later 25 per cent will be fully recovered and 35 per cent will be very significantly recovered and living virtually independently. The question is why does it seem to take so long? Can recovery not be achieved earlier in the course of the disorder? Numerous factors can hinder recovery including stigma, poor concordance with medication, excessive medication, substance misuse, social isolation and lack of opportunity within the community. For carers, friends and sufferers who are starting to glimpse the prospect of recovery this book will give much needed insights and very practical guidance. For those who struggle every day with the distress of unremitting hallucinations, paranoia and low motivation this book may provide techniques to reduce distress and improve quality of life. We need always to be aware of 'red flags' which indicate that we need to reach out for expert's help in the form of a crisis team or emergency department and a number of these 'red flags' are mentioned in the text. Our services are evolving with psychosis pathways being set up which attempt to organise early intervention with personalised care packages delivering evidence based treatment. Cognitive behavioural therapy (CBT) and family therapy are evidence-based treatments which will be considered along with antipsychotic medication which remains the mainstay of effective treatment. The mental health service may decide to deliver low intense CBT techniques or organise for a full course of expert CBT for your family member with schizophrenia. It is important to find out the exact elements of the care that is being organised. You should let your key worker know that you are attempting to deliver CBT informed caring to enhance the treatment being offered. Unfortunately, there are many locations where not only is a CBT or family therapist hard to find but so too is a regular appointment with a mental health professional. This book adds to the others available which attempt to give guidance in the face of under-funded mental health provision. If you do find an approach or style that seems to be beneficial, then do continue to practice and work with it and take advice as to the next steps at your following appointment.

Many gems await the reader in the pages that follow.

Chapter 1

What Is Psychosis? What Is Schizophrenia?

David Kingdon

Key Points

1. Psychotic symptoms can be very understandable.
2. They can also lead to distress and be long-standing.
3. Psychosis covers quite a range of experiences and has a variety of causes.

Why Does Understanding What Psychosis Is Matter?

When unusual experiences or distressing feelings occur, understanding what they are helps in developing confidence and working out what best to do to cope with them.

Life can be confusing at times, stresses can weigh in and motives can be difficult to understand. Sounds can be misheard and strange things seem real but then may fade away. Anybody can make a mistake, but usually we can recognise that mistakes have been made and we can then change our mind. Sometimes though, the belief takes root and seems to be confirmed by other things that are going on. We tend to seek information that confirms what we believe rather than what goes against it, and this can make it even more likely that we hold on to beliefs that may not add up.

It also seems that our mood affects this. So if we are depressed, we think negatively; if happy, positively; if feeling suspicious or unsafe, then what we think fits with that – people are not on our side. We don't talk about being a bit psychotic very often, though often use terms like a 'bit crazy or mad'. With some circumstances, we are a bit 'paranoid' or 'we must be hearing things' might be said. We could be getting a bit muddled or mixed up or getting the wrong end of the stick. It's quite common to mishear things – for example, a humming sound can sometimes take the form of a song or a rustling sound, whispering. A loud noise that startles can even seem like someone shouting. This gets worse when people are stressed, but can also happen when we're just feeling tired and sleepy.

So How Can Psychosis Start?

Quite often it's a gradual process – when we're feeling stressed, a bit unsure about what is happening. We might be feeling a little bit depressed or anxious. Maybe things going on in our lives are making things difficult. We may be feeling bullied at work or at school or generally feel we've been got at. At other times, good things are happening – they can make us feel really good, proud of ourselves, positive about the world and that we have a special place in it. This should always be true to some extent – everybody has a special place in the world, but sometimes it's possible for it to get exaggerated a bit. We might wonder if we are really designed for a very special purpose – to save the world or protect a famous person. Especially if we've been feeling ground down, this can be a really good feeling. This can make us feel really important – and it is important that we feel important – feeling good about ourselves is right. Something can happen to us – something said on the television, radio or lyrics of a song – can lead us to think that we do have a special purpose or mission or ability, and then it sort of sticks in the mind and becomes a particular fixed belief. It may be that when we actually talk about it for the first time, we get quite a positive reaction, but it also can be a negative one, which can either lead us to think 'maybe I got this wrong' or the reverse, that this must be true if people are reacting so strongly. They must have something to hide.

When we talk about someone experiencing psychosis, we are usually referring to our opinion that they are mistaken about what they are seeing, hearing or believing about the world around them. They may be seeing things that, quite simply, other people can't see even though they are looking in the same direction at the same object, or maybe the things being seen are in space but, again, are not visible to others. Commonly these visions come and go very quickly, but sometimes they can be more persistent and can then be quite frightening and distressing.

More commonly, people can hear things that others don't hear or don't interpret in the same way. For example, the rumble of thunder might sound like the word of God or the hum from the fridge may be a repetitive command to harm us. On other occasions the sound may seem to come completely out of the blue with no stimulus at all. Although sometimes this can be sound which has no meaning, usually these experiences do have meaning; they sound like speech, and things said are more often negative than positive. Sometimes they can be positive – they can be complimentary, they can be reassuring and sometimes be the voice of somebody who has been a support to us in the past, for example, a grandmother or teacher.

But voices are more usually neutral or negative when related to psychosis and sometimes say things that have no meaning whatsoever. They sometimes just reflect what we have been thinking; they might even be like an echo of what we've been thinking. They can be quite unpleasant, especially if they are telling us to do things or are swearing at us or telling us how bad we are. Often what is said is something that has been said to us before by someone who has been in a powerful position over us. So this might be a father, stepfather, mother, teacher, care home worker or a boss at work. The memory of those things that are said can come out very vividly, as a voice. When something has a strong emotional association, like something said, but also something that happens to us, like a serious car accident, the experience is etched on our memory so it is very easy to recall or for something that is associated with the event to trigger it. This trigger can be a word, sound, smell or something we see.

Suspicion is also something that can develop into a psychotic symptom. It is reasonable to be suspicious of people we don't know and to be careful about how much we trust them. It's actually very important that we aren't too trusting because people unfortunately can be deceitful and take advantage of us. Whilst most people probably wouldn't do this, it's nevertheless important that we develop relationships before we put our trust fully in somebody. It is reasonable not to trust strangers unless there is a good reason to do so – for example, we would probably trust a bank manager or doctor because of their status, but not somebody we had met for the first time in a pub or on a train. They might seem very pleasant and trustworthy, but first impressions can be wrong. However, this can go too far and because we've been taken advantage of or bullied, we can end up not trusting anybody and develop the belief that everybody is against us. When we break it down, think it through, it usually is only a particular group of people we have reason to be suspicious of and generalising to everyone, or almost everyone, can interfere with life significantly. We talk about people becoming paranoid in this instance. Again it is important to be sensible about who we trust, but it's also reasonable to accept people's positive motives if they've demonstrated them and not to expect them to be out to get us when the evidence really doesn't add up to that. Sometimes there may be particular reasons why we might feel that people in general have got it in for us, but it's really important to work this through and take a balanced look at whether this is the case or not. Specifically, it is worth trying to work out what it is that leads us to believe that people can be trusted or not. This includes governments, employers and other organisations.

Sometimes these beliefs about other people can take the form of feeling that they are trying to control us. There is, of course, some degree of truth in this – governments, police and others do have power and influence over us, but they should use this according to the laws that we, as a society, agree to and give them. They certainly shouldn't use it in a way that picks out an individual unfairly. Also, it is possible sometimes to believe that they have special powers and ways of controlling us involving surveillance or technological devices. Certainly it is known that organisations like the CIA, MI5 or the Russian secret service have in the past experimented with all sorts of devices to manipulate people, but not a lot of evidence that they have been successful in this yet, and even in these circumstances, there is generally some control exerted by government, and the uses to which these powers are put will be related to national security. Certainly the use of such powers with civilians seems very well controlled – or at least that is what most of us believe. If we think otherwise, it's important to work through the reasons why and what benefits there might be for an organisation, such as government, in trying to control an individual who is not in a position to threaten national security. Why should we be picked out? What makes it worth investing lots of time and resources in surveillance or control of us?

It's also possible to believe that our thoughts might be controlled or that thoughts are being put in our mind, perhaps by some sort of telepathy or mind control. Telepathy is interesting, and there are a lot of descriptions of twins, for example, being convinced that they can communicate feelings and thoughts. There have also been experiments to try and demonstrate that it is possible to transmit thoughts between people in separate places, but the evidence isn't very good that this is possible. Similarly mind control sounds possible, at least in science fiction films, but again there doesn't seem to be any clear scientific evidence that this can happen. People can strongly influence others, but the idea that the mind can be controlled or movements controlled by an external force again is interesting, but there seems to be nobody who is very clearly claiming and demonstrating they can do it. If we think it is happening to us, it can be very worrying, but there doesn't seem any evidence that it can happen.

Another common and distressing thought is that people can know what we're thinking – they can read our minds. That is particularly distressing if what we're thinking at the time is something we might be ashamed of or feel guilty about. Our mind responds to all sorts of things going on and triggers in the environment – things we see or hear – and so thoughts that are sexual or violent or just strange come and go very easily. Usually we just let them pass and don't pay too much attention to them, but if we feel they are being broadcast to other people, as it were, that can certainly be distressing. But again this sort of telepathic transmission may happen in the movies, but there is no evidence that anybody has been able to make it happen in real life. What can happen is that we recognise somebody is feeling upset, distressed or happy in response to something they are thinking or is happening around them. The way they react, their expressions, movements and 'body language' can tell you a lot about what they feel, but that's different from being able to have our thoughts read.

What about Thought Disorder and Negative Symptoms?

Another event that we talk about as being related to psychosis is that thoughts can get jumbled up ('thought disorder') or perhaps, more accurately, the way they are communicated, how they are spoken, can seem unclear. This can mean that people seem to be making jumps from one topic to another without it being clear what the link is, or sometimes they seem to be saying things that don't make sense, using words that seem to be made up of other words put together. This can get quite confusing and make people wonder what the person is trying to say. Again this can happen in other circumstances where we don't even think of psychosis. Some people do tend to talk in a way that can be difficult to follow, although they may be very clear about what they mean. If we stop them and ask some questions, they can explain this – and this is actually exactly the same with people when we talk about them having 'thought disorder'. So thought disorder is really just an exaggeration of speech that is a bit garbled and difficult to follow. We often find that someone who is speaking in a way that is difficult to understand is understood by family members or friends who know them.

Another group of problems needs to be considered. When we're feeling stressed and anxious, a common response is to withdraw and get away from the stress. If we feel people are talking negatively about us or are getting at us, again a simple way to deal with that is to avoid seeing people and, similarly, if we feel they are interfering with our thinking in some way. But this can then mean that we get isolated and it can be difficult to get back into meeting people again. Stress can certainly worsen voices and the way we feel in general, so avoiding stress is quite natural. All this can be quite demoralising and depressing such that we feel less and less likely to do anything. And if we don't do anything and don't go out that becomes depressing and we get into a vicious circle rather easily. If we feel criticised, it's quite natural not to say much, and we can seem to appear more and more blank and expressionless to others. We can also end up speaking less and less, especially if we are not seeing people very often. These ways of reacting have been described as negative symptoms but are really about reacting to circumstances which can be difficult and where avoiding stress makes sense, at least in the short term. The problem is that in the long term it limits our lives very significantly and can stop us doing the things that we want to do in life like developing relationships, being independent and doing things that can be interesting and productive.

The other things that can happen with psychosis include being depressed, anxious, obsessed and confused; having sleeping problems or eating problems; and being angry and frustrated. All these can be reactions to what is happening but also problems in themselves that can be helped.

How Common Are Psychotic Experiences?

The best attempts to look at this have been through surveys of people in their own homes. These have sampled populations with interviewers literally knocking on doors asking people about what they feel, their experiences and what they do. They've used screening questionnaires to ask about experiences that seem to relate to psychosis and then followed these up with more detailed interviews where appropriate. There are, of course, problems with such surveys, and people who are particularly withdrawn or suspicious are less likely to respond, answer the door and agree to an interview, so it's likely that these methods underestimate the number of people in the population who do suffer from psychosis. Some surveys (e.g. in Scandinavia) have added other routes to identify people with psychosis, such as using housing department, hospital and general practice records. From these surveys it looks likely that at any time 15 to 20 per cent of people are having experiences that are like psychosis and that perhaps 3 to 5 per cent are experiencing psychotic symptoms, but these are not necessarily persistent and tend to come and go. Then maybe 1 per cent of people or possibly more have beliefs that have been in place for quite a while and who can benefit from help. This is the end of the spectrum of psychotic experiences which is given the label of schizophrenia.

What Causes Psychosis and Schizophrenia?

A number of things seem to make it more likely that people will have beliefs and experiences that are related to psychosis. These include using illegal drugs such as cannabis, amphetamine and cocaine, although this is not the case with opiates – heroin or morphine. It does seem that when people move house or country, this can make them more vulnerable, and there is something about being the second generation whose parents have moved to the country and then had children, who then seem to be more vulnerable. It's not at all clear why this happens and may have something to do with feeling rejected by that society, especially through experiences of racism. Poverty and living in a city also make psychotic beliefs more likely, and there is some relationship with levels of intelligence, but it remains the case that anybody can develop psychosis – you can't be too clever for it. This has included Nobel Prize winners in the past.

Childhood experiences also seem to be very important for many people who experience psychosis. There is now a lot of evidence that physical, sexual or emotional abuse in childhood makes people much more likely to develop mental health problems, including psychosis, but it is also the case that many people who have such experiences can live happy and fulfilling lives. It's also the case that even where the experiences have caused distress, it is still possible, with help, to learn to cope much better with them, recognise that they are not at fault for what happened and move on with their lives.

Psychosis is a very broad set of conditions, and the reasons why it develops varies. The events that happen to us interact with our family upbringing and the genetic coding that comes from our parents. Genes undoubtedly affect areas such as our appearance and our personality. These are very important in the way that we respond to the world and the world responds to us. For some people, traumatic events or drug use do not have a major effect on them, as they have a degree of resilience that, along with the circumstances they find themselves in, protects them. For others this can lead to them becoming confused, suspicious and seriously affected in terms of the way they feel about themselves and about those around them. Also it is possible, because of the way we've grown up, we may have been relatively isolated or bullied and therefore become more suspicious and detached from the world. This can mean that when things do go wrong, suspicion can turn into paranoia and beliefs develop that people are against us.

Cultural beliefs can also lead to confusion, as many beliefs held by different societies and cultures are appropriate for one but seem strange or irrational to another. This has led to considerable problems in assessing whether somebody has psychosis and is a very important consideration now whenever an assessment is being made. Family members, friends and community leaders can be incredibly helpful in deciding when somebody has appropriate cultural beliefs or when it has gone beyond what is normally the case.

So suspicious and confusing beliefs are pretty much universal, especially when we are stressed; psychosis involves experiences that have developed past this into paranoia, thought disorder and hallucinations (hearing voices or having visions), but these are less common – they can become very distressing and get in the way of living our lives. This is the subgroup of people with psychotic experiences who carry the diagnostic label of schizophrenia. Understanding these experiences and discussing them can make a big difference.

Personal Disclosure

Hearing voices is a very common experience and one which I remember occurring when I was a teenager on one specific occasion when I'd been watching TV one evening. I heard my mother shout 'David', startled and then realised that she was not in the house. What I heard sounded completely real, but could not have been from her despite it being her voice.

There have also been times when I have been very suspicious of others and their motives, especially in relation to being turned down for grants or publication – not necessarily being paranoid but certainly having the feeling at times that others around you do not have your best interests at heart. Of course, I might be right about that, but probably in retrospect, it was possible – maybe even probable – that the grant applications or papers simply weren't good enough!

Example

John had worked in a large firm but gradually became more irritable, difficult and angry. It took a long time for him to express what the problem was, but in an outburst one day, he accused his employers and work mates of ganging up on him and making his life a misery. It took time to explore why this belief had developed, but it traced back to a number of years before when the system of appraisal within the firm had changed and after getting good appraisals, his assessments became much more average with some criticisms of his performance. He ruminated on this and eventually came to the conclusion that this was related to a conspiracy targeting him. Discussion with him reduced his level of distress and allowed him to re-engage with his family, and the beliefs themselves reduced in intensity over time.

Complex Example

June presented with distress, self-harm and anger. She was actively hallucinating and was very paranoid. The voices she heard were of her brother threatening her and God telling her to kill herself. She was very fearful of others and isolating herself, but repeatedly presented to emergency services with self-harm. Work with her enabled her to understand the relationship of the voices to abusive experiences in childhood, but work on these experiences and the beliefs about herself required sustained support from a multidisciplinary team, crisis planning and therapeutic involvement over a number of years.

Further Reading

Emotional wellbeing site (information about mental health). https://emwb.org.uk/

Freeman, D. Freeman, J. & Garety, P. (2016) *Overcoming Paranoid and Suspicious Thoughts* (2nd edition). Hachette, London.

Gumley, A. & Schwannauer, M. (2006) *Staying Well after Psychosis: A Cognitive Interpersonal Approach to Recovery and Relapse Prevention*. Wiley, London.

Hayward, M., Strauss, C. & Kingdon, D. (2012) *Overcoming Distressing Voices*. Hachette, London.

Longden, E. Learning from the voices in my head (TED talk). www.ted.com/speakers/eleanor_longden

Morrison, A. P., Renton, J. C., French, P. et al. (2008) *Think You're Crazy? Think Again*. Routledge, London.

Mueser, K. & Gingerich, S. (2006) *The Complete Family Guide to Schizophrenia*. Guilford, New York.

Romme, M., Escher, S., Dillon, J. et al. (2009) *Living with Voices: 50 Stories of Recovery*. PCCS Books, Manchester.

Psychosis Usually Has a Natural Tendency towards Recovery

Thomas Christodoulides

Key Points

1. 'Psychotic' experiences such as hearing voices, holding beliefs not held by others and feeling paranoid are all much more common than we might think.
2. These experiences are usually an understandable reaction to what's happening in our lives. Often factors like sleep deprivation, trauma, isolation, substance misuse and stress are precursors.
3. For most people, psychotic experiences are often brief and do not cause any major disruption or distress.
4. Even when these experiences are more prolonged, many people live with them without any negative impact on their lives. In fact, many people value these experiences, feeling that they have learnt something from them, that they enrich their lives and that they have helped them in some way.
5. For many, however, these experiences can be frightening and can have a devastating impact. However, even with a chronic history, some degree of recovery is the most common outcome.
6. Lastly, what do we mean by 'recovery'? It means different things to different people. In other words, it's a journey that is defined by the individual themselves.

Introduction

In this chapter we will explore the notion that for many people 'psychotic' experiences, such as holding unusual beliefs or hallucinating, are brief, do not necessarily have a negative impact and can even provide an enriching experience. Of course, this may come as a surprise to many others for whom such experiences are scary, confusing and overwhelming. It begs a key question: What can help us understand, cope and even thrive with psychosis? Later in the chapter, two case studies will be described, each illustrating some Cognitive Behavioural Therapy (CBT) techniques that can aid recovery in those struggling with experiences like these.

Psychotic Experiences as a Common Part of the Human Condition

Hearing different voices in our heads is a normal part of the human experience, widely accepted throughout society and not a sign of mental illness at all. According to Julian Jaynes, author of 1976's *The Origin of Consciousness in the Breakdown of the Bicameral Mind*, this was how we humans viewed voice hearing before 1300 BC, before we coined the term 'consciousness'. For those who hear voices, Jayne's theory can be an attractive one. It provides a reassuring message: that hearing voices does not mean you are ill or different. It also raises a potentially helpful implication too: after all, if these are entirely natural experiences for a human being, can this provide us with a clue about how we cope with them?

It was in 1987 that Jayne's work took a more public turn. Two Dutch researchers, Marius Romme and Alexandre Escher, invited one of their patients onto a television chat show in Holland. Patient X was a voice hearer who spoke of Jayne's work and how helpful and reassuring he had found it. After being interviewed on the television, a request was put out for other voice hearers to get in contact. They were inundated. Of the 450 voice hearers who got in contact, 150 people reported being able to cope with their voices. Although initially startled and frightened by the initial presence of a voice, people had a range of understanding about their experiences, and many felt they were not ill or disabled by them at all. Coping seemed to align with some accommodation of the voice as part of themselves. According to Jayne, this may be how we all viewed such experiences pre-1300 BC.

It is not only voice hearing that we can view as a natural and common part of the human condition. It seems that feeling unsafe and paranoid is also commonplace. Freeman and Freeman provide examples in their 2008 book 'Paranoia': Did you know that 40 per cent of UK adults believe that 14 is the earliest age at which children should be allowed out unsupervised? It's not just that we are feeling less safe; we also feel less trusting of authority. For example, nearly 50 per cent of people in New York believe that the terrorist attacks of 9/11 were known about in advance and deliberately ignored by US leaders. The proportion of people who believe in phenomena that have not been scientifically validated is also striking, with many polls reporting high proportions of people believing in ghosts, unidentified flying objects and extrasensory perception. Of course, the vast majority who hold these beliefs are not 'unwell' or unduly distressed by them. In fact, many would say that they take pleasure from them and that they don't interfere with their daily lives. Likewise, studies have shown that many find voice hearing to be valuable, helpful and enriching, providing companionship, comfort and support. For example, nearly 50 per cent of the 'good copers' who contacted Romme and Escher in response to the television programme saw their voices as a 'special gift'. Many famous, successful and artistic people experience voices or delusions too. Modern examples include Anthony Hopkins, John Frusciante (guitarist from the Red Hot Chili Peppers) and Nobel Prize–winning mathematician John Nash (made famous in the film A Beautiful Mind)'. An older example is Charles Dickens. He famously heard the voice of Mrs Gamp, from his novel Mrs Chuzzlewit. She would tell him rude stories in church, making him laugh out loud! It also seems that culture can make a big difference to how we view hallucinations and unusual beliefs. For example, a number of Amazon tribes, such as the Cashinahua, view hallucinations positively, as phenomena that help guide them on a spiritual journey.

Personal Disclosure

Missing My Train

A few years ago, I was asked to represent the northeast contingent of the British Psychological Society at their national meeting in London. The meeting was at 10 a.m., meaning I had to catch the 6 a.m. train from Newcastle upon Tyne. I slept in, missed my train and arrived at the meeting, oh only about four hours late! I rather sheepishly introduced myself to my colleagues and promised myself I'd never let this happen again. Skip forward three months to the next meeting. Well, this time, I set three alarms and swore I'd make my morning train! Trouble was, I was so anxious, I didn't sleep at all. I made the train, the meeting went fine, and I travelled back north later that day on a very busy connection. As I sat there, feeling pretty exhausted, I heard the train hospitality attendant ask me, 'Tea?' 'Yes please,' I replied, 'milk, no sugar'. I turned around, but no one was there! Everyone was staring at me, somewhat concerned. What had happened? I looked again to check, but again, no one was there, and I was now only attracting more looks. As I sat in my chair, I quite frankly panicked. But then gradually I began piecing it together: I had just experienced a brief hallucination, sometimes referred to as a BLIP (brief limited intermittent psychosis).

Questions

1. What factors do you think may have led to my BLIP?
2. How common are BLIPS like this?
3. What was it about the experience that made me panic?

In hindsight, it's clear to me that my levels of stress and lack of sleep had made me exhausted. We all know that we're not at our best when we're stressed and tired, but did you know that this is also when our perception can become 'fuzzy', often leading us to have odd ideas and brief hallucinations? These BLIPs are actually incredibly common: just ask any sleep-deprived new parent or night-shift worker. Why did I panic though? Perhaps because I didn't have a frame of reference for what was happening to me. In our Western culture, we don't speak of these experiences, and they are often stigmatised, associated with mental illness, hospitalisation and words such as 'mad'. Contrast my hallucination with another reality-bending experience that we all have: dreams. Dreams are so powerful, strange and feel so real at the time. Yet most of us are able to experience them nightly and get on with daily business without a second thought. How? Maybe, in contrast to hallucinations, modern Western culture views dreams as understandable, acceptable and even enriching parts of the human experience.

Question

How would we feel and cope with these experiences if our culture viewed them as common and understandable as dreams?

So far we've seen how psychotic experiences are common, often fleeting and can be manageable and viewed positively. But what can help recovery if they are more frequent, distressing and prolonged? Let's learn from two examples of recovery, based on real service users' stories (anonymised and amalgamated to protect confidentiality). First, the story of a young man who entered an early intervention in psychosis (EIP) service, troubled by voices.

A Simple Example

James was a 17-year-old young man who lived with his mum and dad and two older sisters. They were a close and supportive family, who regularly attended church together. Over the previous six months, James had felt under tremendous pressure to do well at his upcoming exams. He was revising every night until late and worrying all day that he wouldn't get the grades to get to a top university to study medicine. This had begun to badly affect his sleep, as he was lying in bed worrying for hours, sometimes sleeping as little as one to two hours at night. He began to hear the odd voice, but it quickly escalated into hundreds of times per day. The voice didn't sound like him, said horrible things and threatened to hurt his family. He was very scared of the voice and worried that it was a demon, one so powerful that it could hurt his family.

Questions

1. What factors might have contributed to James hearing voices?
2. Why did he find these experiences so distressing?
3. What might recovery look like for James?
4. How likely was recovery for James?
5. What do you think would help James recover?

As we have learnt, James' example is more common than you might think. We also now know that certain conditions make it much more likely to hear voices, for example, lack of sleep, stress, trauma, substance misuse, prolonged isolation and sensory deprivation (*see the 'Links' section at the end of this chapter for a link to a YouTube clip that illustrates this*). For James, he appeared to be under tremendous stress, and his sleep was severely disturbed. Had he also been isolating himself to concentrate on his studies? Also, this was not just a single stressful day but had been going on for a prolonged period. James reported that he found his experience scary, which is a common reaction and understandable; after all:

- the voice was saying nasty things and making threats
- he felt that it was very powerful and could harm someone close to him
- he thought that it was a demon
- he had no other explanation for what was going on
- he did not know how to cope with it
- he was already under a lot of stress and hadn't slept well

When something happening to you is so scary, it can be hard to see how things can get better. But did you know that recovery is very common for people in James' situation? About half of us will experience problems like this on one occasion and then will recover completely (Cooke, 2017).

There is no one accepted definition of recovery. It is an individual's journey, meaning different things to different people. So, it was important for James to define this for himself. He stated that he wanted an explanation – why was this happening to him? He also wanted to be rid of the voice. If that wasn't possible, he wanted to be able to get on with his day without it bothering him. Let's look at his first steps.

An Alternative Explanation

James was offered help in an EIP service. His therapist began by developing an alternative explanation of what might be going on here. Perhaps this was not a demon at all, but maybe this was a common reaction to too much stress, severe sleep deprivation and James isolating himself in order to study. James was dubious, but through looking at lots of information together, he slowly began to think that perhaps there was something in this (*what information did they look through? refer to the 'Additional Reading' and 'Links' sections at the end of this chapter*).

Table 2.1 Behavioural experiment template

Belief	Test	Prediction	Outcome	What was learnt
The voice can carry out its threats if I don't respond	Challenged the voice to knock a picture off the wall	It will do it (70%)	Nothing happened	Maybe the voice isn't as powerful as I thought

Power

Often voice hearers report that their voice feels very powerful and that this is one of the most distressing aspects of it. This was the case with James; his voice was making threats to harm his family if he didn't say certain phrases back. The therapist and James used a 'behavioural experiment' technique to test the power of the voice (*a template is provided in Table 2.1*). James picked a low-level threat that it made and for once, he tried not responding to it. When nothing bad happened, he repeated this and then expanded it to other threats. After a while, James felt confident that he could challenge the voice and even dared it to carry out tasks that he put to it – e.g. 'if you're so powerful, make that picture fall off the wall in the next two minutes'.

Alternative Coping

After some time, James felt his belief in the voice's power began to drop, and he was left with a question: 'If I don't need to obey it, what should I do when I hear it?' The therapist and James tried a technique called 'leaves on a stream' *(there is a link to a script in the 'Links' section at the end of the chapter)*. Lots of practice with this technique helped James distance himself from his experiences and let his voices 'be' without responding or trying to change them.

Helpful Aspects of James' Experiences

Finally, the therapist and James looked at James' lifestyle that had contributed to his voice-hearing experiences, and he considered if he wanted to keep living this way. Over a number of sessions, James reflected on what was important in his life and decided to work towards a balance between work, relaxation and connecting with others. He decided on limiting his revision time to finish at 8 PM and to give himself two nights a week and one day off at the weekend. He also eased the pressure he put on himself to get all top grades in his exams and began spending more time with his friends and family doing things he enjoyed. Once he had eased the pressure on himself, he began to worry less and his sleep improved. Gradually, James realised that he was in recovery. His experiences hadn't gone away but bothered him far less and didn't interfere with his values or goals in life. Later still, James reflected that the voice-hearing experience was a valuable one and had enabled him to learn a lot about himself. It had shown him his limits and that things couldn't continue the way they were. He felt that his voice hearing was the catalyst enabling him to create a more enriched, connected and valuable life for himself.

James' recovery story is a common one, but sometimes recovery can seem a long way off, or even impossible. Let us look at how recovery was achieved with a more chronic and complex presentation.

A More Complex Example

Luke was a 42-year-old man who lived on his own at home. He grew up in a difficult family environment, with a verbally and physically abusive father. He also experienced many years of bullying during secondary school. He had a number of jobs in the past but unfortunately had not felt able to work or study for the past 10 years or so. His immediate family lived close by, and he saw his mum every week. Luke had felt paranoid for over 20 years and had been hospitalised on three occasions during times when he was struggling to keep himself safe. He had long-standing beliefs that he was being monitored by a sinister government agency, who had bugged his flat and implanted devices in his body. He had cut himself to check for 'bugs' when he had 'felt them under his skin'. He spent most of his time in the flat alone, as he felt that agents were everywhere when he left the house. He felt that they gave off signs that they were following him by looking at him and by sending messages on their phones when he walked past. He had spent a lot of time on his own trying to figure out why this was happening to him but had not come up with an answer. In the meantime, he had lost contact with his friends and was struggling to know what he wanted from life.

Now let's return to the same five questions as before:

1. What factors might have contributed to Luke's paranoia?
2. Why did he find these experiences so distressing?
3. What might recovery look like for Luke?
4. How likely was recovery for Luke?
5. What would help Luke recover?

Luke's experiences were most likely rooted in his earlier life experiences. After all, he felt threatened at home and at school for many years, so it's not a great leap that he had developed a view of the world as threatening and viewed himself as vulnerable. His isolation, although understandable, would have exacerbated his sense of danger from the outside world. Luke's anxiety and coping are actually understandable in the context of his beliefs. After all, wouldn't any of us feel scared if we believed we were being monitored, bugged and followed everywhere we went?

Recovery can seem like a long way off for someone like Luke, who has been hospitalised multiple times and has such a long-standing history. But actually, only a minority of people experience ongoing difficulties like this (Cooke, 2017) and they often gain huge benefit and support from services. Let's see where he started.

Reconnecting with Values

Luke was offered help in a community treatment team. The first step was identifying his strengths and helping him reconnect to his values that are so often disrupted by chronic paranoia. He was referred to an occupational therapist (OT) who completed an assessment, identifying that he valued studying, spending time with his family, learning new skills, building and working with his hands and learning about science. Luke had lost touch with many of these aspects of his life gradually over the past 20 years as paranoia had taken a tighter grip on him. He felt that he couldn't re-engage with activities in line with these values whilst his paranoia was so intense, so Luke was referred to a cognitive behavioural therapist for further help.

Table 2.2 Helpful and unhelpful aspects of coping strategies

	Helpful	Unhelpful
Thinking about 'why is this happening to me?' (rumination)	• Might get to the bottom of it • It feels safe	• Takes up a lot of time • I don't seem any closer to the answer • Sometimes it makes me feel worse
Staying in the house as much as possible (avoidance)		
Looking out for signs that people are looking at me and checking their phones (hypervigilance)		

Considering Pros and Cons

The cognitive behavioural therapist and Luke began by looking at the pros and cons of his current coping with his paranoia. Broadly his coping broke down into three categories: spending a lot of time thinking 'why me?' (rumination), remaining in the house alone (avoidance) and looking out for signs of people looking at him and checking their phone (hypervigilance). Over a number of sessions, the therapist and Luke looked at each strategy in turn to examine helpful and unhelpful aspects of each (*Table 2.2*).

Exercise: In Table 2.2, helpful and unhelpful aspects of rumination are completed. Can you complete the rest?

Testing It Out

After some time, Luke could see that his coping strategies were understandable but came with considerable downsides. He was then willing to look at alternative ways of approaching his paranoia. As the OT assessment had revealed that Luke was keen on science, the therapist tried to appeal to the researcher in Luke. They planned out behavioural experiments to test out different 'hypotheses' about his paranoia (*see Table 2.3*). For example, they sat in a café where people couldn't see them from the street and counted how many people looked at their phones whilst walking. Luke soon realised that everyone was at it, and without being able to see him! This gave him the confidence to test other ideas using this method.

Exercise: Can you design an experiment to test some of Luke's other ideas in Table 2.3?

Seeking Support

After some time, Luke understood that there were different ways to cope with his paranoia, including reinvesting in activities that were important to him. In practice, this was still overwhelming for him, so he was referred to a 'peer support worker' (PSW), a clinician with lived experience who could relate to Luke's situation. Luke didn't feel able to return to full-time education or work, but with support, he felt enabled to seek out, apply and attend a 10-week course in model building at a local college. From this, his confidence grew, and he enrolled in more online courses and began spending more time with his family. His paranoia remained, but his beliefs about his paranoia had shifted. If people were monitoring him, he didn't want it to stop him leading the life he wanted anymore. After some time, Luke was asked to share his recovery experiences with other service

Table 2.3 Behavioural experiment template

Belief	Test	Prediction	Outcome	What was learnt
People look at me and check their phones because they are monitoring me	Observe how many people look up and check their phones when they can't see me (for 30 minutes)	People won't be looking up and checking their phones (60%)	People looked up/checked phones 56 times	Maybe this is something everyone does and is not about me
If I think about 'why this is happening to me' for long enough, I'll get the answer				
I can't get any joy from any of my old hobbies anymore				

users, to speak at local conferences and to help contribute to service developments within the team that had once helped him.

Helpful Aspects of Luke's Experiences

Luke's experiences were chronic and devastating with multiple admissions to hospital and enormous disruption to his wellbeing and functioning. However, the experiences had also enriched him in some ways. Given his past, Luke had learnt something extremely valuable: he now understood that safety would most likely always be very important to him but that it need not define every aspect of who he was. Given his life experiences, he had also learnt to acknowledge how resilient he had been to cope for so long and how much stronger he must be to have thrived in the circumstances. His experiences also enabled him to share his journey with others, gaining a sense of satisfaction and value from teaching and helping.

In this chapter, we have seen that psychotic experiences are common, are often brief and that many people feel enriched by them. The stories provided examples of journeys to recovery w hen the experiences were troubling and even chronic. We finish with some CBT tips to remember, some additional reading and finally some links to recommended web material that elaborates on this chapter.

Summary of Key CBT Techniques: Dos and Don'ts

Do ... consider alternative explanations for the experiences. Have poor sleep, isolation, trauma, substance misuse or stress played a part?

Do ... consider pros and cons of your coping strategies.

Do ... keep testing out different ideas or ways of coping with your experiences – either on your own or with the help of a clinician.

Do ... try to keep a focus on your strengths, values, roles and goals in life. Bear in mind that these experiences do not have to define you.

Don't ... go through this alone. Sources of support can come from your friends and family, your community, local National Health Service (NHS) and volunteer services and self-help books, as well as websites and online forums.

Don't ... forget some key messages from this chapter – these experiences are very common, often in reaction to difficult life circumstances, and recovery is the most common outcome.

References

Cooke, A. (Eds.). (2017). *Understanding psychosis and schizophrenia: Why people sometimes hear voices, believe things that others find strange, or appear out of touch with reality, and what can help* (2nd ed.). Leicester, UK: The British Psychological Society Division of Clinical Psychology.

Freeman, D. & Freeman, J. (2008) *Paranoia: The 21st century fear.* Oxford: Oxford University Press.

Jaynes, J. (1976) *The origin of consciousness in the breakdown of the bicameral mind.* Boston, New York: Houghton Mifflin Company.

Further Reading

The following books offer CBT self-help techniques to help work towards recovery:

Freeman, D., Freeman, J. & Garety, P. (2006) *Overcoming paranoid & suspicious thoughts: A self-help guide using cognitive behavioural techniques.* London: Constable & Robinson Ltd.

Hayward, M., Strauss, C. & Kingdon., D. (2012) *Overcoming distressing voices: A self-help guide using cognitive behavioural techniques.* London: Constable & Robinson Ltd.

Morrison, A., Renton, J., French, P. & Bentall, R. (2008) *Think you're crazy? Think again: A resource book for cognitive therapy for psychosis* East Sussex: Routledge.

Turkington, D. et al. (2009) *Back to life, back to normality: Cognitive therapy, recovery and psychosis.* Cambridge: Cambridge University Press.

Links

The following websites/links illustrate and expand on themes within this chapter: www.intervoiceonline.org/ is the international hearing voices network website which provides positive messages about hearing voices, including articles on recovery and an online community forum.

www.paranoidthoughts.com/ provides a paranoid thoughts questionnaire, personal accounts of paranoia and advice about coping with paranoia.

www.ted.com/speakers/eleanor_longden Eleanor Longden talks about her recovery journey with an encouraging message for those who hear voices.

www.youtube.com/watch?v=0nnekxGE0nM is a four-minute YouTube clip that demonstrates how quickly hallucinations and paranoia can be induced in anyone within 48 hours.

www.bps.org.uk and search for the 'understanding psychosis and schizophrenia' PDF, which offers a comprehensive overview of the current state of knowledge in the field.

www.mindfulnessmuse.com/wp-content/uploads/2011/09/Cognitive-Defusion-Exercise-1.pdf offers a script to use for the 'leaves on a stream' exercise.

Links to Other Chapters

More examples and discussion of positive experiences of beliefs are available in Chapter 3.

Further advice on techniques that can help with recovery are illustrated in Chapters 5, 7, and Chapters 12–14.

More detailed examinations of particular experiences such as 'delusions', hearing voices and visions are provided in Chapters 9–11.

Positive Aspects of Psychosis
Enhanced Spirituality and Creativity

Maggie Douglas-Bailey

Spirituality in simple terms is 'consciousness'. All living beings have levels of consciousness that allow reasoning, logic, growth, qualitative knowledge and interaction to occur. The quest for knowledge and reason varies from person to person, creating varying levels of spirituality/consciousness.

On a humanistic level, we can communicate and understand each other, whereas on a higher level, some seek to find reasons for our presence on earth, how we got here and/or if there is anything outside of this plane. To be able to access these other planes, individuals require entrance to a different level of consciousness, which requires being vulnerable or 'psychically open' (Grof & Grof, 1987). From birth, all living creatures are 'psychically open'; for example, children have imaginary friends. In African and Asian societies, however, this 'psychic openness' is welcomed and nurtured from childhood and viewed as a powerful gift.

Adapting to Western cultural and societal expectations, we explore ways of managing our 'psychic openness' to avoid being stigmatised and isolated, thus making it dormant through the life span. This openness is simply waiting for a chance in some people to be reopened. This usually occurs on re-experiencing a 'psychic surge' (Warwick, 2007). This could occur after an emotional challenge, which leaves us seeking answers (why are we in so much emotional pain, feel the way we do, etc.), for example, after a relationship breakup or death.

Spiritual mediums and psychics claim to be able to access a different plane of consciousness, where they are able to see colours, faces, shapes and occurrences; to predict the future; understand the past; and confirm the present to bring peace, hope, understanding, proof, comfort and support to others.

One significant difference between mediums, psychics and people with schizophrenia is that spiritual mediums and psychics are thought to harness this level of consciousness through prayer for protection and creative expressions. They also manifest it through their use of language in their teachings in churches of their experiences, poetry, imagery, drawings and 'open circles' (where messages are given to others). It is very clear within mediumistic and psychic practises that messages of hope, comfort and support are relayed to the congregation and not ones of pain, loss and distress, which seem to be present within schizophrenia.

Creativity within schizophrenia has also been of comfort and a useful outlet for the reduction of the distress experienced within schizophrenia.

This chapter outlines the links between spirituality (mediums and psychics) and schizophrenia and ways of coping through creativity.

Personal Disclosure

As a young child, I always felt there were others that neither I nor other people could see around me. I did nothing about this but was often afraid to be alone. I and everyone else around me also noticed that I was extremely 'sensitive' to other people's feelings – I could feel other people's pain and anguish (particularly that of strangers) and would often express them to my grandmother, who was always ready to normalise while nurturing my experience. Being outgoing, it was often easy for people to speak with me and vice versa, thus explaining and informing strangers of what I could feel had happened or what was going to happen to them. This was usually accepted, particularly in a culture where children are often seen as having spiritual gifts.

Along with this spiritual gift I was also very creative. I wrote poetry, musical lyrics and sang. As I got older and lived in the United Kingdom, I learned to ignore the feelings, thoughts and presences.

At 25 years of age, after a relationship breakup, I found myself in a spiritualist church, where I was informed of my 'gift of foresight and empathy' (I did not believe it!) and was even more shocked when I stood up and began to inform one of the senior mediums of the death of her child, providing her with details that only her family was aware of. She confirmed and validated my proof of evidence and thanked me. I felt strange, as I did not feel that I had done anything. However, the proof that there is life after this life and the existence of a higher power seemed to be very comforting to those present. I strangely felt like a huge weight had been lifted off my shoulders. I noticed that by attending the church and working as a medium, I felt lighter, less stressed and happier. Then I soon noticed a feeling of being strangled at night and a darkness coming over me, and I became scared. Struggling with understanding it all, along with my mother's belief that what I was doing was wrong, I no longer attended the church. After a few months, I began feeling very ill, having sleepless nights with nightmares, became paranoid and began obsessively checking things – doors, cookers, lights, cleaning, etc. – things I would usually not be too concerned about. I asked the spirits to leave me alone, but they wouldn't.

I returned to church after a while, explaining this to the other mediums who explained, 'Now that you have accepted your sensitivity, you have to protect yourself from other entities through prayer and imagery'. I learned how to cope. I practised with imagery and prayer and proceeded with my work at the church and returned to 'normal'. I could sleep again, the obsessive behaviour ceased and I was myself again! I have come to recognise the burning feeling in my heart when something is about to happen to someone I am close to – the only problem is that I am unable to tell who or what is going to happen.

In the beginning, I genuinely thought I would have to be admitted to a psychiatric hospital with this experience, but I was supported by more experienced mediums, and these gifts became easier and clearer. I now have very vivid dreams about certain situations. I must admit that I have so far not been able to do anything to change the situation or forewarn the individual. I have, however, been able to support them afterwards.

I can see (sometimes on flooring, walls etc.), hear, feel and sense 'spirit'. I am able to contain these experiences to certain times of the day or even week. I make time to communicate with them and protect myself. I have never been diagnosed with schizophrenia or any other mental health condition (I do not believe I have a mental illness). However, I am aware that had I gone to the doctor with my symptoms, I would have been diagnosed with psychosis or something similar.

Lessons Learnt

1. Everyone experiences distress in different ways.
2. Everyone is potentially 'psychically open', for example, hearing your name being called out and not seeing anyone around.
3. Culture and society create a stigma that eventually creates the term 'schizophrenia'.
4. With support and comfort, all spiritual experiences can be positive.
5. Creativity is required as an outlet for spiritual experiences.

Exercise

1. Ashley was sitting and suddenly thought of her friend Aaron. She had not heard from him for a while. She thinks of contacting him and is distracted. Soon after, the phone rings. Ashley answers the phone, and Aaron is on the other end.
   This is the uncanny experience of synchronicity and can be seen as the universe informing you that you have done something right.
   Have you ever experienced something similar?
2. Malcolm is busy mowing the lawn, but his mind is worrying about his ill daughter; he hears his name being called, he turns around, but there's no one there. Have you ever experienced this? In this case there are three possibilities: a misperception of a voice though white noise, a hallucination due to stress/vulnerability to psychosis linked to worry or a spiritual warning. Often, the last possibility isn't even considered.

Spiritual Voices and Schizophrenia: Toni's Story

As a child, Toni had an imaginary friend (Ralph) whom she was very close to. She was always on her own and spent little time with others in the nursery, but she was very popular at school. She informed people of what was going to happen before it did. Initially, people thought she was strange, but others thought she was brilliant!

However, at 16 years of age, Toni was involved in a car accident that took the life of her aunt, with whom she was very close. She was angry and stressed. Toni was no longer able to utilise her skills, which led to her being bullied at school. Soon after, she lost her parents. Struggling, Toni became paranoid, seeing faces and animals, hearing negative voices (which scared her) and struggling with life in general.

Diagnosed with depression and on the verge of being sectioned, Toni felt even more isolated, as there was no improvement in her symptoms and no one to help. In a dream, Ralph appeared, giving her encouragement and hope.

Ralph urged her to remain positive, get up, get dressed and live life. Toni eventually gained the courage and did just that. A few weeks later, Toni, with Ralph's encouragement, found her way to a community centre, where she began telling others her story. One of the ladies (Gloria) understood what she was experiencing and asked if she could spend time with her and share her story with other sufferers.

With both Ralph and Gloria, Toni continued sharing her story and helping others. She gradually became better with no more negative voices or images. Toni is now helping others with similar experiences.

There is hope in this world.

Spiritual Voices and Schizophrenia: Complex Case – Adam's Story

Adam comes from an extended family of people who could hear, see and feel things and tell the future and past. It was evident that Adam shared this gift. However, his Roman Catholic parents, who shared the same gifts, had fought against these gifts of seeing and hearing 'dead people'. They prevented Adam from nurturing his gifts even as a child. However, the rest of the family (grandparents, aunts and uncles) were positive and encouraged him to embrace and nurture his gifts.

Adam's parents soon forbade him from doing so and prevented him from associating with the rest of the family. Adam was devastated! A few weeks later, Adam became withdrawn, detached, stressed and depressed. His parents kept praying for him, but he had lost interest and motivation for everything. He was paranoid, scared and kept talking about being watched, threatened and potentially being killed by people his parents could not see, hear or believed existed. Two months later, Adam was worse. He was not washing, eating or speaking with his parents.

They contacted a doctor, who diagnosed Adam with schizophrenia. Ashamed and unable to help their son, Adam was eventually admitted. On hearing of Adam's predicament, his grandparents began visiting him in hospital. After a while, Adam began responding to his grandparents, talking to them about what was happening to him.

They gradually nurtured, worked, guided and taught him to protect himself. Two years later, Adam understood the importance of protecting himself, managing his health and affording time to the spirits to help others.

Adam's parents are still not accepting of Adam's beliefs but are very happy that their son is well.

There is hope!

Voices in Spirituality versus Schizophrenia

Some of the differences between voices heard in schizophrenia and by a medium are listed in Table 3.1.

Table 3.1 Differences between voice hearing in spirituality vs. schizophrenia

Spirituality/mediums	Schizophrenia
Inside and outside ear	Inside and sometimes outside ear
Provide validation/proof	Commanding
Calming voices	Harsh
Provides support and comfort	Brings fear and discomfort
Encourages writing/drawing	Discourages writing/drawing
Use of imagery	Not enabling imagery
Encourages communication	Isolating
Listens to the vessel/individual	Creates fear
Is patient, caring, loving, compassionate	Intrusive, repetitive, can appear caring but often isn't
Soothing/protection	Bullying/destruction

Worry Associated with Spirituality and Mediumship

The stigma associated with having different experiences often leads to worry, stress and fear for both the carer and individuals involved. Hearing your loved one report such symptoms will usually elicit worry in carers. Worry can lead to several severe health conditions. It is therefore important to deal with worry quickly and appropriately.

CBT techniques for worry:

1. Talk to someone about your concerns.
2. Write down your concerns clearly and honestly.
3. Look at the positive and negative aspects of your concerns.
4. Look and see what you could do to change the situation.
    a. If you can do something about the situation, then do it!
    b. If nothing can be done about the situation, let it go.
    c. This could be done through:
        i. Visualising yourself letting go of the worry
        ii. Meditation
        iii. Burning a letter and releasing it into the air.
5. Devise a worry tree, mapping out how, when and what can be done about your worries. This way, you have a plan of what can be done if those circumstances arise.
6. Allocate time to worry (say 15 minutes each day). In this time, worry as much as you possibly can.

Positive Aspects of New Belief Formation

Mediums and psychics have similar experiences to people with schizophrenia, which involves, seeing, hearing and feeling things that others don't. These experiences, when nurtured, can be expressed creatively. For example, Jesus Christ heard, saw and felt others' pain and could express this through his teachings, miracles and empathy. Van Gough, despite his psychotic experiences, could make fabulous artistic breakthroughs in his paintings. Another example is Anthony Hopkins; despite hearing voices, he was able to forge a very successful career as an actor.

Conclusion

The ability to express oneself through creative channels, such as spirituality, imagery, music, art, acting, writing and dancing, is essential, as it provides an outlet for releasing emotions. Support, effective communication and shared experiences in groups are essential if one is to avoid psychosis as these gifts begin to emerge. Perhaps a more detailed exploration of spiritual mediums' and psychics' experiences and coping mechanisms may be beneficial in understanding of the symptoms of schizophrenia and ways of better coping with them. CBT for people with psychosis needs to embrace the issue of 'psychic openness' and ask questions relating to spirituality and creativity at the time of assessment. During the formulation period of CBT, such elements need to be endorsed as strengths and unique aspects of their personal and symptom development. Personal disclosure could facilitate improved collaboration, and the normalising of such experiences could act to reduce stigma. Later in therapy creative imagery is extremely useful in working with negative emotions, and creative writing as homework can aid in the recovery process.

References

Grof, S. & Grof, C. (1987) Spiritual emergency: The understanding and treatment of transpersonal crises. *Re-Vision*, 8, 7–20.

Warwick, S. L. (2007) *Psychic opening as spiritual emergence(y) and its relation to self-defined seeking*. Unpublished Masters Thesis, Liverpool John Moores University.

Further Reading

Clarke, I. (2008) *Madness, mystery and the survival of God*. Winchester: 'O' Book.

(2010) *Psychosis and spirituality: Consolidating the new paradigm*. Chichester: Wiley.

Fletcher, P. C. & Firth, C. D. (2009) Perceiving is believing: A Bayesian approach to explaining the positive symptoms of schizophrenia. *Nature Reviews Neuroscience*, 10, 48–58.

Useful Websites

Spiritualcrisisnetwork.uk
www.mentalhealthforum.net

When Can Psychosis Escalate and Will Medicines Help?

Douglas Turkington

Key Points

1. Psychosis can become more severe or entrenched due to the emergence of frightening beliefs about the symptoms; using safety behaviours such as social isolation; or becoming depressed, ashamed or sleep deprived.
2. A person is less likely to recover from psychosis when self-treatment is used in the form of cannabis, legal highs or hallucinogens such as amphetamine, cocaine or LSD.
3. About 25 per cent of those with escalating psychosis will have a really good response to the first antipsychotic medicine taken. If a response is going to occur, there will be clear signs of progress with two weeks, if concordance is good. Many others respond but to a lesser degree.
4. A further 25 per cent of those with more entrenched psychosis will respond to clozapine, which has a different mechanism of action.
5. Stopping and starting antipsychotic medicines is bad for the brain. It is really important to take the agreed amount regularly. Do not stop taking the medicine suddenly; schedule an appointment so that a gradual reduction in dose can be attempted with support.

Introduction

We have seen that hallucinations and paranoid thoughts are common human experiences and that the human cortex can easily produce these symptoms under certain conditions of stress. Usually these symptoms are limited and persons recover once the stress is reduced. A case example will clarify this point. Li was a 32-year-old high school teacher. Due to staff sickness and annual leave, he had to cover extra duties and became increasingly distressed and developed a degree of insomnia. Li started to have problems concentrating and developed intrusive thoughts of losing control and being violent in class. He had never had such thoughts before and started to wonder if these thoughts were being beamed into his mind by a local extremist terrorist group. Li was encouraged to visit his general practitioner, and when he disclosed his ideas, he was deemed to be suffering from schizophrenia and at high risk to others. Li became increasingly stigmatised and started to consider suicide. He was seen by an early intervention psychiatric nurse, who was able to explain that the violent thoughts were just intrusive thoughts, which were very common in people under stress. The nurse showed him Rachman's list of normal intrusive (obsessive) thoughts and explained that people hardly ever acted on them. Li started to manage his stress and worked on improving his sleep pattern. He let the violent thoughts come and go and stopped catastrophising about them. The nurse was able to explain to him that he didn't have schizophrenia, and the diagnosis was changed. The whole matter was explained to the school, and Li returned to work. This was a narrow escape – how many people have gone down this pathway into a wrong diagnostic label and a lifetime of distress, unnecessary medication and social decline? However, schizophrenia does exist and can most definitely need medication. Schizophrenia, which is mostly caused by genetic or biological factors or triggered by illegal drug use, is most responsive to antipsychotic medicine. The traumatic subtype of schizophrenia is less responsive to medication. Similarly, the type of schizophrenia which manifests with a bizarre delusional system and grows from deep roots within the personality is also less responsive. A very thorough psychiatric assessment is the first port of call, and to be honest, this cannot be done in less than two hours and a collateral history from the family is a crucial component. Such a thorough assessment is critical to decide when to start a trial of medication. Remember the story of Li – the assessment allowed a low-intensity CBT intervention to obviate the need for medicine in his case.

Personal Disclosure

Having developed a degree of asthma (does everyone have asthma nowadays?), I was prescribed a Ventolin inhaler to reduce bronchospasm and a Becotide inhaler to prevent bronchospasm. I seemed to be fine taking Ventolin as often as needed (particularly if the temperature suddenly dropped) but seemed to avoid taking the Becotide inhaler, which would have prevented the wheezing all together. I am a medic! I know how they work! Concordance with medicine is a very individual phenomenon. After 20 years of this pattern, I eventually realised that I was wakening at night due to nocturnal asthma and this was causing fatigue. I eventually started to take my medicine properly and to my benefit. What do you think explains this phenomenon? I think in retrospect that I needed an expert to spend more time with me, who could have explained more about the illness and its treatment. I also think I needed to accept it more as a real factor in my life and not something that could just be swept under the carpet. How many people with schizophrenia are taking the same approach as me? I am now much better!

So what can we conclude?

1. Concordance with medicines needs to be individually assessed.
2. We should never presume that the medicine is being taken as prescribed.
3. If a person is not adhering, then there will be a good reason which can be explored.
4. Concordance interventions are almost never done.

Positive Aspects of Medicine Use

Lina had a delusion of persecution. It was triggered by overwork and cannabis use. Unfortunately, the first medicine she tried caused weight gain and sedation, and she stopped taking the medicine suddenly but felt too ashamed to tell anyone. The psychosis deteriorated, but she did start to strike up a rapport with the crisis team and disclosed the problems with the side effects. Lina was offered a choice of a range of different antipsychotics and she chose one that was weight neutral and nonsedating. She was much better at taking these and made an excellent recovery. So a prescriber can engage the patient in selecting their antipsychotic based on preferred side effect profile. This can greatly enhance concordance and therefore outcome. Similarly, some people would prefer to choose a weekly, fortnightly or monthly injection, which gets rid of the need for daily medication reminders.

Self-Treatment with Cannabis

Bob quite definitely derived some benefit from antipsychotic medication but still had symptoms of persecutory paranoia and delusions of reference from the television and radio. These symptoms left him with anxiety and ongoing worry and rumination. Instead of finding out more about the delusions and testing them out with the help of his best friend Joseph, he stayed at home and smoked up to a dozen joints every day. He swore by the cannabis – Bob believed that the cannabis was an effective treatment, as it made him feel 'chilled out'. When considering the pros and cons of 12 joints of cannabis per day, Bob agreed that over the years of this practice he had steadily lost motivation to do anything outside of the home. He also agreed that his concentration and memory were less good than before. Bob agreed that it was possible the cannabis haze was even making the paranoia worse but in a chilled-out way. It was also costing him a fortune to keep his habit going. The big pro seemed to be the benefit on anxiety. So the pros and cons, when listed, seemed to point towards the need for activating an effective anxiety reduction measure, CBT to investigate the delusions and begin to test them out and a gradual reduction in cannabis. Bob came off cannabis with the use of mindful breathing exercises and anxiety-reducing medicine. He then worked with Joseph to list other possible explanations of his delusions and test these out.

Clozapine Can Be a Miracle

Brian had received numerous different antipsychotics but had always declined the offer of clozapine, as he didn't want to have blood tests. He had been ill for 18 years with voices, a delusion of demonic persecution and negative symptoms. Clozapine was started as a last resort, and although it took about three months to work, Brian made dramatic progress in all of his symptoms. He was happy to put up with the side effects of sedation and some weight gain to have much of his old lifestyle back and his symptoms markedly controlled.

Simon's Relapse

Simon became thought disordered and had somatic hallucinations and negative symptoms following a period of increased socialisation and pressure at work. He made a full recovery with his first antipsychotic, and this was supplemented by expert CBT. His family was fully informed and had access to the audio files of the therapy. Some crucial relapse prevention advice was provided and discussed several times. First, don't overdo it socially or in terms of getting back to work. Second, keep regular hours and maintain activities and report any early warning signs to family members and to the key worker. Last, this medicine has really worked – Simon will need to take it regularly for at least two years and then may consider a very gradual reduction in the dose. After two weeks of feeling really well, Simon went out to an all-night party, applied for a job in Brazil, returned to his work full time and stopped his medication. He relapsed over the next two weeks and soon he was thought disordered, preoccupied, behaving bizarrely and not caring for himself. He agreed that the medication could be restarted. It didn't work the second time around and neither did any other antipsychotic or clozapine. Stopping and starting a medicine is a bad strategy that almost always triggers relapse. If a person is determined to stop a medication, they need to tell someone first and book an urgent appointment so that psychiatric input and increased support can be provided.

Conclusions

Antipsychotic medicines can deliver a very real recovery for many people but sometimes don't fully work and CBT and other strategies are needed. Review the side effects of the different antipsychotics and request your choice. Ask for a trial of clozapine if you are no better after a year. Consider the case examples in this chapter and consider reducing or stopping cannabis. Don't stop and start antipsychotics. Always seek psychiatric help if attempting to reduce the dosage and do so gradually.

Links to Other Chapters

Chapter 5 shows how frightening explanations, worry, rumination and social isolation can perpetuate psychosis.

Making Sense of Psychosis

Helen M. Spencer

Key Points

1. It may be difficult for service users and carers to make sense of the symptoms of psychosis.
2. Psychotic symptoms in schizophrenia are better understood through the process of developing a formulation.
3. There are different types of formulations, such as the A-B-C model, which is written in a linear form; the maintenance formulation, which is often represented as a self-perpetuating cycle; and the timeline, which looks back over the person's life history.
4. A formulation diagram outlines an event and how an individual then responds to that event in terms of their thoughts, feelings and behaviours. However, these ways of responding might actually be keeping the problem going and maintaining the symptoms of psychosis.
5. Drawing out a formulation diagram is a joint process between the service user and therapist, who try to work together as a team to understand and make sense of what is happening. This type of guided discovery can lead to dramatic breakthroughs in understanding the psychosis and the reason(s) why it has developed for the person at this point in time.
6. Carers and friends can get involved by helping the individual to draw out formulation diagrams as part of homework in between the therapy sessions.

Introduction

It can be very confusing and baffling for carers, family and friends to understand what is happening to their loved one when they start to experience psychotic symptoms for the very first time. Indeed, it can be a very strange and frightening experience for the individual themselves, who may ask family and friends 'Why is this happening to *me*?' and 'Why now?' In schizophrenia, service users and carers very often become paralysed by this question because they just can't make sense of what is happening.

In CBT, the therapist's aim is to work with the service user by helping the person make sense of their unusual experiences. This joint or shared process also seeks to make sense of why the symptoms developed in the first instance, what is keeping them going (or maintaining them) and what can be done to better manage these symptoms or get rid of them altogether. In CBT this 'making sense' process is referred to as a formulation and is often represented in a diagram. Making sense of experiences via the use of a formulation is a joint process where the service user and therapist work together as a team. Ultimately the formulation can help guide and inform treatment; therefore, it is a crucial step to allow change to occur.

This chapter outlines what carers, friends and service users can do themselves to make sense of the psychosis by using simple formulation processes.

A-B-C Formulations

An A-B-C model or formulation (Ellis, 1957) shows how thoughts, feelings and behaviours may be linked together, for example, in relation to voice hearing (Figure 5.1):

In other words, the **A** (Activating event) triggers the **B** (Belief) that the person believes to be true, which leads to the **C** (Consequences). In this example, the **A** refers to a person hearing a critical voice. Following this experience, the emotional **C** is feelings of anxiety and sadness. The behavioural **C** might then be social isolation, or even self-harm.

As a therapist or carer, we can help the person make sense of the **B** – what are the thoughts or beliefs that the person has about these voices? In this example, it would be 'the voices are telling the truth, I am a failure'. This, of course, can be worked with in CBT by looking for evidence of this presumed sense of 'failure' and coming up with some alternative, rational responses to what appears to be a global unrealistic belief.

Another A-B-C formulation, for example, in relation to a persecutory belief, may look something like this (Figure 5.2):

The **A** would be the activating event: seeing a police car drive past the house. The **B** would be the delusional belief itself: that the police are looking to arrest and imprison the person for no real reason at all. The emotional **C** would be severe anxiety and guilt, and the behavioural **C** would be to find a safe place to hide at home. Here the A-B-C helps to make sense of symptoms that appear to be puzzling and complex by mapping them out in a simple diagram. Once we have made sense of the psychosis in this way, the next step might then be to ask the service user to make a diary record of how often police cars drive past his house: is this excessive or the same as in other nearby streets? Are police cars really driving by as often as he thinks and, if they are, could there be an alternative explanation (i.e. is there a police station nearby that they are driving to and from?).

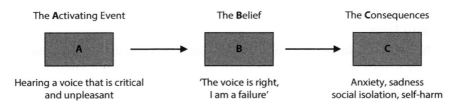

Figure 5.1 An example of an A-B-C formulation for voice hearing.

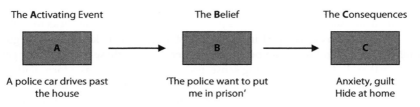

Figure 5.2 An example of an A-B-C formulation for a persecutory belief.

Maintenance Formulations

The symptoms of psychosis are often made worse by feelings of panic, shame and self-stigma which often develop alongside 'safety behaviours' as people try to keep themselves safe and manage the frightening symptoms as best they can; for example, listening to loud music may be used as a safety behaviour as an attempt to try to 'drown out' the voices. Or the service user might close all of the curtains in the house in an attempt to prevent government or terrorist surveillance. Unfortunately, these safety behaviours, although understandable as a response to certain beliefs, are not always the best means of coping and can often make things worse or exacerbate symptoms and perpetuate an ongoing vicious cycle. This process can be represented in a diagram which CBT therapists often refer to as a maintenance formulation (Figure 5.3):

In psychosis, a maintenance formulation (Morrison, 2001) like the one shown here, is often presented in a circular diagram which helps to show how certain thoughts, feelings, physical reactions and behaviours (or ways of reacting to an event) can actually maintain the problem and keep it going in a way that is difficult (but not impossible) to break. If we refer back to the person with critical voices, we can see how 'safety behaviours' such as listening to loud music can make the person feel on edge and hypervigilant, and lying awake all night can lead to sleep deprivation – both serve to maintain the experience of hearing voices.

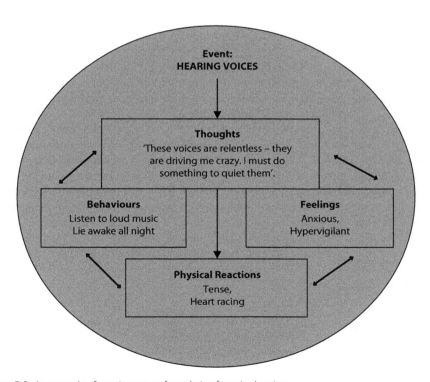

Figure 5.3 An example of a maintenance formulation for voice hearing.

Timeline Formulations

One of the most crucial questions in making sense of psychotic symptoms is to ask 'how did this all start?' and 'why now?' Timeline formulations can help the person trace their history by going back to the start and discovering that there was a trigger (or multiple triggers) in the person's life history that can help to explain why their symptoms developed in the first place. Timeline formulations can then help to normalise these symptoms based on triggers or past life events, such as a family history of schizophrenia, a traumatic life event, childhood abuse, bullying, excessive stress and many other factors that may have resulted in the 'tipping point' that pushed the person too far. In CBT, the person can learn that each and every one of us could develop psychotic symptoms if we were pushed to our limits.

Positive Aspects

Timeline formulations can be positive if they can also help the person recognise their areas of strength and resilience, instead of just highlighting all that is wrong with them (Kuyken et al. 2009). For example, how have they managed to cope with the stresses and strains of life so far? What are they good at? And what areas of strength can they draw upon now to help them cope better with this particularly difficult time in their lives?

Because of the complexity of the timeline and the emotions that may be unearthed, for example, in relation to trauma disclosure, it is advisable to explore the timeline with an expert CBT therapist and not attempt to do this on one's own or with a family member or friend.

Personal Disclosure

Some unusual experiences such as voices or visions can also be positive in nature, and it can be helpful to try to make sense of them in terms of a formulation. Soon after my own grandmother died following a long terminal illness, I was reading through an old birthday card that she had given me some years ago. On the front of the card there were some butterflies, and inside the card she had wished me a happy birthday and had also written 'fly with the butterflies'. When I read this, I felt a mix of emotions and I cried and laughed at the same time! At that moment I saw a butterfly fly slowly and gracefully past me. The butterfly was right in front of my eyes and it was white and transparent. I did not see it enter my visual field and I did not see it leave. It was a strange experience, but when I think about my timeline, my grandmother had always enjoyed watching the butterflies in her garden, and each summer we used to watch them together when I was younger. Seeing a vision of a butterfly seemed to have personal meaning and was very reassuring and comforting at the time. It certainly helped me through the grieving process.

A Simple Example

I am a perfectionist and procrastinator. There I said it! I tend to put off important jobs, as I worry that I'm not going to be able to do them 100 per cent perfectly. I had critical and unforgiving parents. The harsh criticisms conveyed to me as a child became my own inner self-talk. The way in which my parents spoke to me became the way that

I began to relate to myself in my own mind as an adult. So the criticism continued, like the parents I could never get rid of! In line with this, I tend to put off important jobs in case I am criticised by others. This, of course, can be very frustrating for my colleagues, who may feel the need to criticise me for not having finished important jobs! Anxiety and sadness are the typical emotional components on my formulation. So now that I have understood myself better, I can make sense of my situation. Can you see how my maintenance and timeline formulations fit together? But how can I use CBT to change all this? Writing down and challenging my critical and perfectionist thoughts would be a good place to start, as well as learning to develop a more kind and compassionate way of relating to myself so that I can allow myself to be imperfect and to do a job that is 'good enough' (Gilbert, 2010).

A More Complex Example

Gemma had very critical voices which escalated in intensity until she self-harmed. The more she was criticised by her voices, the worse she felt about herself and the more she self-harmed. Her self-harming required crisis team intervention, and a hospital admission was looking increasingly likely. In terms of the A and C these were straightforward, but what was Gemma's belief about her voices – the B? Gemma was telling herself that the voice was a ghost which was very knowledgeable and very powerful.

It was clear that something needed to be done to reduce the self-harm, to make it less frequent and less dangerous. So the CBT aimed to develop better coping strategies to replace the self-harm, as well as working out some alternative explanations: was the voice really an intelligent and powerful ghost? Perhaps in our CBT session we could test its knowledge by asking it some general-knowledge questions such as 'What is the capital city of Albania'? Or we could ask the ghost to demonstrate its powerfulness by moving the coffee table across the room. Gradually using psychoeducation along with these exercises, Gemma began to realise that voices are very common and not as clever or as powerful as she had once thought.

In time, Gemma became more assertive; she stopped self-harming and reclaimed her life. There was, however, a timeline formulation here which helped to make even more sense of her situation.

Gemma had well-meaning parents who actually wanted the best for her but perhaps did not realise how critical they were being during her adolescence. The message Gemma received was often 'you are just not good enough, there many things about you that are flawed, why can't you get out of bed and get a job? You are just lazy'. Gemma left home as soon as she could and set up in an inappropriate relationship with an older man who, of course, criticised her and eventually became physically violent. So the A-B-C, maintenance and timeline formulations all helped to make sense of the psychotic symptoms that presented, as well as highlighting several different treatment options. Like my own example of my internal critical thoughts, Gemma also needed to learn to self-nurture and to show compassion for herself, to soothe the critical voices that bullied her. There are a variety of homework exercises within CBT which can be done to develop self-compassion, as well as the use of effective techniques as seen in compassion-focussed therapy (Gilbert, 2010).

Summary of Key CBT Techniques: Dos and Don'ts

Do ... help your loved one to make sense of their experiences using the A-B-C and maintenance formulations.

Do ... try to keep formulation diagrams simple.

Do ... use guided discovery and find things out together.

Don't ... attempt timeline formulations without a CBT therapist.

References

Ellis, A. (1957) Rational psychotherapy and individual psychology. *Journal of Individual Psychology*, 13, 38–44.

Gilbert, P. (2010) *Compassion focussed therapy*. London: Routledge.

Kuyken, W., Padesky, C. & Dudley, R. (2009) *Collaborative case conceptualization: Working effectively with clients in cognitive-behavioral therapy*. New York, NY: Guilford Press.

Morrison, A. (2001) The interpretation of intrusions in psychosis: An integrative cognitive approach to hallucinations and delusions. *Behavioural and Cognitive Psychotherapy*, 29(3), 257–76.

Additional Reading

Irons, C. & Beaumont, E. (2017) *The compassionate mind workbook: A step-by-step guide to developing your compassionate self*. London: Robinson.

Websites/Other Info

treatingpsychosis.com

Links to Other Chapters

Chapter 6 on trauma, Chapter 11 on visions and Chapter 12 on compassion-focussed approaches.

What If the Psychosis Is Linked to Trauma?

Lucy H. Stevens

Key Points

1. Trauma is something that can happen to anyone; it is not a defined event; rather, what the event means to us is of most importance.
2. Traumatic experiences have been linked to psychosis, where evidence is strongest for childhood abuse, and risk of perceptual experiences such as hallucinations (hearing, seeing, feeling, smelling and/or tasting things others cannot).
3. Unusual beliefs and perceptual experiences can form to protect us from uncovering the nature, or experiencing the pain of, an earlier trauma.
4. Memories of traumatic experiences are stored in our brain and body, which can lead to persistent feelings of fear and threat in the present, regardless of the outcome of the traumatic event and our ability to consciously recall it.
5. Fear and anxiety can change the way we think about things and heighten our senses, which can make us vulnerable to 'psychosis', as this involves more extreme changes in perceptual experience and the way we think.

Introduction

What do we mean, as professionals, when we are talking about trauma? The word trauma perhaps implies somewhat mystical properties, almost as if it is distant from reality and involves certain adverse events that do not happen to 'normal' people. These include experiences that are abhorrent, totally horrific and render the person completely hopeless to the horror that is unfolding in front of them. This is a myth, of course, as traumatic experiences are more common than we may think and they can include a range of different events. Although our reaction to such events (i.e. the intense feelings of horror and helplessness) may be true in part, it is much more realistic to open our mind to trauma and think of these experiences as occurring on a continuum. Many events may occur on the continuum of trauma, for example, losing a job, getting a divorce, financial difficulties, up to more extreme forms of abuse and torture; all of these can be viewed as being potentially traumatic for some people, but what defines this as being traumatic or, rather, a difficult life event is the meaning this holds for the individual and how that meaning and the trauma affect the person's life. Given that we are all individuals and have different values and experiences in life, we know that what one person may experience as being very difficult may be different from one person to the next, so we should never assume to limit trauma as being related to particular events.

An example of an event that tends to divide opinion in society is retirement. Retirement can be a very positive thing for some people. I know my father very much enjoys his retirement and days spent on the golf course! However, I also know people who have viewed retirement as a loss and experienced a range of negative feelings, such as feeling sad or guilty as a result of having more time to evaluate and look back on life; feeling de-skilled, useless and even inadequate; and experiencing a loss of identity or role in society. All of these feelings are equally viable in response to retirement and can increase someone's vulnerability to experiencing difficulties adjusting. Therefore, even a life event such as retirement that is routine, part of most people's lives and is very positive for some people can have the potential to be traumatic for others.

What does trauma have to do with psychosis then? There are many different ways in which the aftermath of trauma can influence our thinking, perception and behaviour, and is a subject that is too broad to be covered in entirety in this chapter. A good starting point is to ask yourself, 'what has happened to me?' rather than 'what is wrong with me?' A lot of research is beginning to suggest that there is a link between traumatic experiences and the subsequent distressing unusual experiences that are often seen in psychosis. For example, a study by Kim Mueser and colleagues (Mueser et al., 1998) found 98 per cent of 275 people suffering from severe mental illness (including psychosis) had experienced at least one traumatic event, and Romme and Escher (1989) found that 70 per cent of people connected the onset of voice-hearing experiences to a threatening/traumatic life event. The research is a bit of a minefield, so I will not go into too much detail here (I will try and keep it brief!), but a list of useful resources and websites is provided at the end of this chapter that you can view yourself should you wish to do some further reading.

Traumatic events during childhood have been highlighted as particularly important. When talking about these types of experiences, these are indeed experiences that would be interpreted as traumatic for most people; there is less research investigating the role of general life events (such as retirement), as these are so individual it would be very difficult to draw any conclusions! Childhood abuse (emotional, physical or sexual) and neglect (emotional or physical) have been the most researched, with the suggestion that these experiences carry the highest risk for developing psychosis. For example, studies as a whole have suggested that people with psychosis are more than twice as likely (2.7 times) to have been subjected to childhood abuse than other people in the population (Varese et al., 2012), and this risk increases if we are subjected to more than one type of abuse, if it is prolonged and severe, if it occurred at a younger age and if it was perpetrated by someone close to us such as a parental figure (e.g. Fisher et al., 2010; Janssen et al., 2004; Read et al., 2003).

We believe these experiences are important because when we are younger, experiences help shape our developing brain and belief system, which enables us to feel safe in the world. For example, if someone close to us or someone in a position of trust hurts us physically, such as a teacher, neighbour, babysitter or family member, it makes sense that we may be wary of that person in case this happens again. When this happens on multiple occasions, we may begin to wonder if any adult we come into contact with may pose a physical threat. As a result, we might learn that it is always important to remain guarded and mistrustful of others to keep ourselves safe, as our fight/flight alarm system is telling us we have experienced pain and harm before and we must be careful. It is easy for this belief to become quite fixed as our alarm system is telling us 'better safe than sorry'. However, sometimes our carers and parents may also feel a sense of blame for not being able to keep us safe, and this can make things difficult for them and us, as it is not always possible to protect a child from traumatic experiences. An example of how neglectful experiences could affect us is if a responsible adult has not looked after us and given us the care we needed, such as a teacher or babysitter, whom we may spend a lot of time with, being dismissive when we are upset; we may hear the voices of others or see others who are not there as a means of feeling some sense of love, care or safety in a lonely world. However, voice-hearing experiences can sometimes take the form of the perpetrator of abuse or become distressing for many other reasons, and this is when we would consider these experiences as a symptom of psychosis, because voice hearing is prevalent in the population and can remain a functional response to adverse life events.

Trauma can also be related to the formation of unusual beliefs, which we may refer to as delusional when beliefs become very fixed as the person is unable to generate alternative ideas, and this begins to affect a person's life and functioning. Such beliefs can have very protective elements, as a response to trauma. For example, a person may become increasingly religious following a traumatic event, as it may be helpful for them to believe there is a supreme being responsible for their protection. Alternatively, in delusions of persecution, when we view the source of threat as being from other people (e.g. "other people are dangerous or will harm me"), this leads to a natural conclusion around keeping safe, to limit our contact with others and withdraw. Although this is unhelpful in the long- term as we are likely to feel very lonely and isolated, in the short-term it allows us to feel more reassured that we can do something to prevent a bad traumatic event happening again. Sometimes we may attribute a disproportionate amount of blame to the self (e.g. 'perhaps if I had not worn that skirt when I went to meet the man, I would not have been assaulted'), and again, in some ways this can help us to feel safer in the aftermath of a traumatic event, that by changing our own behaviour, it is less likely we will be harmed in the future. All of these examples help us to feel we can lead a 'safe enough' life, through creating some perceived sense of certainty and predictability, but these beliefs have the potential to become difficult and distressing if they persist.

Personal Disclosure

I remember when I was around 16 to 17 years of age, I was at college studying my A-levels, and although I was having a great time, A-level exams and coursework were very stressful. I was also going through the learning curve of gaining and exploring my newfound adult independence! I was someone who was never used to being in the house alone or doing things for myself. I guess you could say I was quite spoilt as a child and rarely left to make my own decisions, so this was a big time for me. I recall entering the house one afternoon after a lecture at college, putting the alarm off in the house, sitting down in my favourite armchair and switching the TV on. After a couple of minutes I started to hear some noises upstairs. I had already been somewhat fearful of being on my own, given that it was not something I was used to, and remember being told by parents and family 'it's just the pipes' when I heard noises. I tried to reassure myself with this, but when the noises started to sound more like distinct footsteps, I felt a real sense of panic set in. My heart started pounding, and I felt frozen to the spot in fear. When I did manage to move, I reached for the telephone behind me and called my brother, who said he was at college, and I also called my great aunt who lived nearby. In the end, my aunt came to the house and told me I was being silly, but when she went upstairs to check the house, someone jumped out at her and gave us both a huge fright. It turned out my brother had been play-ing a prank on me! He told me he snuck in the front door as I was switching the alarm off.

Although the outcome of this incident did not result in a situation that was life threat-ening, the important things to consider are my thoughts and feelings at the time the experience was happening to me. My perception was that I was in great danger. I was experiencing a strong sense of confusion knowing that I unlocked the door and switched the alarm off, but I also felt totally powerless to escape the situation. I recall being frozen in the armchair, listening helplessly to the sounds above. Despite the resolution of this situation and the conclusion that there was no real threat, some of the anxiety around this persisted. For example, when I was alone in the house shortly after this experience, almost automatically I found myself thinking of the experience and having similar thoughts that I had at that time. These thoughts naturally led to some of the physical sensations I described before in the face of no existing threat. When I started to feel this way, I noticed that I was picking up on every sound in the house, and at one point, perhaps even actively listening for noises as a means of checking out whether I was safe or not. Of course, this just made me feel even more anxious because if you listen for noises, it is almost certain that you will hear something!

This example shows how the brain's capacity to pick up on different senses, thoughts and feelings according to our experiences can occur almost automatically. It is a powerful thing, as it is not only the way we think about things that changes, but our actual percep-tions and hence evidence for what is happening changes because the brain does not like conflict. Listening out for things, as I described earlier, is related to something we call hypervigilance, which is a natural outcome of anxiety. However, given this power of the brain to change our thoughts, perceptions and feelings as a result of a difficult experience entering our mind without conscious awareness, it is understandable, if this threat per-sists, how this can transition into starting to hear noises that are not there or that other people cannot hear.

Positive Aspects of the Experience

As silly as it may sound, no matter how extreme and distressing the event(s), we can develop very powerful facets, values and characteristics of the self as a result of hav-ing experienced this. These attributes are so special, that I like to refer to these as 'gifts'. Actively looking for these gifts and values can help us place things in the past instead of longing to change it. Can you think of any gifts a difficult experience has brought you? Some examples people have mentioned may be that this has made them a better and safer parent through perhaps not wanting their own children to experience maltreatment they may have received as a child, feeling a stronger and more resilient person by knowing you are able to fight the tough times and still be here on the other side. If you are interested, the research talks about this a lot and refers to this valuable learning as post-traumatic growth.

In relation to the example provided earlier, I feel the gift this experience brought me is to gain more insight and understanding into anxiety and why this may have happened. Having such an understanding can help stop this from happening again, whereas people who have not experienced this will be going through it for the first time, like I did, and not have the benefits of reflection. For example, I was able to understand that my brain was processing things in a different way and that I was actually just hearing ordinary noises that had always been present. It also helped me to see how strong I am and that I was able to overcome this at a time in my life that was full of change; it has made me kinder to myself and wise to my likes and dislikes as a person, able to build on the former and understand the latter.

A Simple Example

Mary, a 40-year-old lady, has recently quit her job due to stress. Since she has stopped working she has started to experience thoughts and images from the past when she was sexually abused as a young child by her uncle in her home. She is avoiding watching TV or talking to people, as there is a high-profile sexual abuse case in the media, and this makes the thoughts worse and more distressing. She has thoughts that 'I am sad this has happened to other people as well as me'. Mary recently has had a new neighbour move in below her, who has been abusive towards her. For example, Mary said she and other neighbours had heard him shouting abusive things from his flat downstairs, such as 'slut' and 'shut up and stop moving around', which she felt was directed at her. After a few weeks this led to an incident where he tried to sexually assault Mary one day when she was coming back from the shop and returning to her flat. Luckily for Mary, someone entered the building and interrupted this; otherwise, she was convinced this would have resulted in rape. Mary felt so ashamed she did not dare report this to the police, as he also threatened he would assault her again if she did. Around one month after this incident Mary managed to move to a different accommodation but continues to hear his voice. This led to two realisations: that the voice could no longer be real and must be in her head, as this man is no longer in the vicinity, and second, she noticed the voice was also commenting on things she was doing (e.g. she's making a cup of tea) as well as the derogatory things he had shouted to her. It was at this point that Mary presented to the GP for help and was referred to secondary care services for support with psychosis, which is the first time she disclosed the past sexual abuse.

In this case, it is clear Mary has managed to cope by trying to suppress the memory of what happened to her. However, current circumstances mean this has overwhelmed her capacity to cope – a number of triggers match the original trauma. For example, the semantic links between the current events and past trauma include media coverage of a sexual abuse case, attempted sexual assault and emotional abuse by a male perpetrator, perhaps also leading her to feel unsafe in her home, as she did as a child. The subsequent voice Mary hears directly represents the perpetrator of the abuse and begins by directly resembling what he has said to her, before becoming more generalised.

Questions

1. Why have these experiences emerged?
2. What can a carer do to help?

A More Complex Example

Jim, a technical support officer for local educational authorities, has recently been struggling at work as he thinks a powerful being is trying to communicate with him through the computer cables. This means he is spending hours examining all cables in the office and looking up methods of communication and telepathy on the Internet. He has started to believe that perhaps he is especially important in some way and that he has been 'chosen' to receive these special messages and act upon them. Jim describes his upbringing as being relatively normal, but rather deprived. Upon further questioning, it seems he was bullied quite severely in secondary school by older peers and felt like he did not fit in. From this point he reported having very low confidence. Jim began to struggle at work after a male colleague was critical around a major piece of work he was doing for one of the schools ('don't do that you idiot'). He claims to also hear the voice of a powerful being, which he thinks may be God, and this helps to direct him in his work. However, this can become distressing as 'God' has also started to tell him to do strange things like 'urinate on that bin'. Jim states he cannot describe the feeling he gets when he hears this, but finds this overwhelming and has started to scratch himself. When speaking to one of his siblings as part of the assessment, they stated that when growing up they had a babysitter who was 'nasty', and he often came in drunk and did irresponsible and degrading things (e.g. urinating on the floor). They never told their parents, as they thought their story would not be believed. Although the siblings stated that the babysitter never beat them, they wondered if he had beat Jim, as Jim was the only other male. Jim's siblings had observed Jim being hit around the head one night and him fleeing from his room in tears.

In this example, the formation of the belief is less directly linked to the trauma, but has formed as a means of trying to prevent the truth from being uncovered. For example, throughout his life Jim has possibly been treated in a degrading way – by his babysitter and the bullies at school – and this means Jim may have developed very low self-confidence. When he was directly challenged in work, this resulted in strengthening the formation of delusional beliefs to help Jim feel more powerful in a situation that he has experienced previously and been made to feel powerless. However, because this event shares some links with past experiences in terms of how this made Jim feel, this has also resulted in a change in the voices which perhaps partly resemble the trauma memory. For example, telling him to urinate in the bin may directly relate to what his babysitter did.

Questions

1. Why have these experiences emerged?
2. What can a carer do to help?

Exercise: Which of my symptoms might be linked to trauma? What will i do differently?

Think about some of the difficulties your relative/friend might be experiencing.

- Can you see any direct functions of these beliefs, experiences or voices?
- What are these experiences trying to communicate?
- Does this link to anything that has happened in the past in any way?

Despite these difficult experiences, think about the positive aspects of these, as overcoming these surely says something about you as a person and brings you qualities you may never have realised.

- What are the positive aspects of having had these experiences?
- What gifts have they brought in life?

Summary of Key CBT Techniques: Dos and Don'ts

Do ... Show genuine empathy and kindness

Do ... Normalise responses by emphasising the adverse and abnormal nature of circumstances, rather than behaviours, to reduce shame/self-blame

Do ... begin by introducing coping strategies to ensure the person is able to establish their safety and 'apply the brakes' during therapy (e.g. grounding techniques, strategies to deal with unusual perceptual experiences).

Do ... Pre-agree a sign (e.g. raising of a hand) when things are becoming too distressing to enable discussion to stop and to facilitate coping strategies

Do ... Use sensory detail/information, bodily senses, feelings and psychotic phenomena (e.g. hallucinations and beliefs) to elicit details around the trauma once the person is stabilised

Don't ... Immediately suggest symptoms can be linked to difficult experiences without exploring the symptoms first, as spontaneous recollection could increase distress without adequate means of coping

Don't ... Immediately try to challenge thoughts and change behaviours, as these could represent important survival strategies, leaving the individual feeling disempowered with no alternative means of coping

Don't ... Coerce the individual to discuss traumatic or past events without their consent or against their will, as this can lead to re-traumatisation

References

Fisher, H. L., Jones, P. B., Fearon, P., et al. (2010) The varying impact of type, timing and frequency of exposure to childhood adversity on its association with adult psychotic disorder. *Psychological Medicine*, 20(12), 1967–78.

Janssen, I., Krabbendam, L., Bak, M., Hanssen, M., Vollebergh, W., Graaf, R. D., & Os, J. V. (2004) Childhood abuse as a risk factor for psychotic experiences. *Acta Psychiatrica Scandinavia*, 109(1), 38–45.

Mueser, K. T., Goodman, L. B., Trumbetta, S. L., et al. (1998) Trauma and posttraumatic stress disorder in severe mental illness. *Journal of Consulting Clinical Psychology*, 66(3), 493–9.

Read, J., Agar, K., Argyle, N., & Aderhold, V. (2003) Sexual and physical abuse during childhood and adulthood as predictors of hallucinations, delusions and thought disorder. *Psychology and Psychotherapy: Theory, Research and Practice*, 76(1), 1–22.

Romme, M. A., & Escher, A. D. (1989) Hearing voices. *Schizophrenia Bulletin*, 15(2), 209–16.

Varese, F., Smeets, F., Drukker, M., Lieverse, R., Lataster, T., Viechtbauer, W., Read, J., van Os, J., & Bentall, R.P. (2012). Childhood adversities increase the risk of psychosis: a meta-analysis of patient-control, prospective- and cross-sectional cohort studies. *Schizophrenia Bulletin*, 38(4), 661–671.

Further Reading

Ainscough, C. (2000) *Breaking free: Help for survivors of child sexual abuse*. London, UK: Sheldon Press.

Romme, M., Escher, S., Dillon, J., Corstens, D. & Morris, M. (2009) *Living with voices: 50 stories of recovery*. Herefordshire, UK: PCCS Books LTD.

The British Psychological Society (BPS) (2014) *Understanding psychosis and schizophrenia* – available from the BPS website

Websites/Other Information

It is important to only access information if you are feeling able and confident to do so. Ideally, this should be done in the presence of a therapist or health care professional or supported by a close other you can trust, such as a carer, family member or friend. However, if you wish to seek support or additional resources please visit:

- Eleanor Longen, health care professional and academic, but also someone with lived experience who gives a very insightful talk on her story of unusual experiences – search for Eleanor Longden TED Talk on YouTube.
- The Hearing Voices Network is a great resource containing information on hearing voices, and they also have a number of affiliated groups set up around the country that people can attend – www.hearing-voices.org

- The NSPCC website contains resources and contact information to receive support if you have been a victim of childhood abuse or neglect – www.nspcc.org.uk

Links to Other Chapters

There are lots of different reasons for the development of psychosis, so it may also be useful to look at Chapter 5. It is important to be compassionate toward ourselves when we have experienced trauma, so a useful chapter would be Chapter 12. See Chapters 9, 10 and 11 for more detail on the unusual experiences discussed in this chapter (e.g. unusual beliefs, hearing voices, seeing things others cannot see).

The Five Pillars of Caring for Psychosis

Latoyah Lebert

Key Points

1. Optimise work/life/caring balance and introduce flow activities.
2. Improve the emotional tone at home.
3. Activate self-nurturing.
4. Use effective communication.
5. Introduce befriending sessions.

Introduction

To develop an optimal caring milieu, the five pillars need to be built; caring doesn't come naturally and needs to be constructed. This chapter will guide you through the five pillars of caring through a series of exercises; a few weeks should be set aside in order for you to practice these techniques.

Personal Disclosure

In my early career I worked as an activity coordinator in a care home. I often found myself spending substantial amounts of time at home after work preparing activities for residents so that I would have more time to spend with them during my working day. There would be a sense of guilt and feelings of inadequacy in my role if I spent my time preparing for activities rather than 'doing' them with residents. These habits then began to affect my personal life as 'me time' gradually decreased and relationships with others I cared about were neglected. I started missing gym sessions, felt tired and as a result gained weight and in turn felt miserable. My work/life/caring balance was out of sync and needed to be corrected. I turned things around by taking up mindfulness techniques and gaining some control of life by returning to gym classes. Slowly taking time to do the things I enjoyed gave me the motivation to find more balance.

So what can we conclude?

1. Sometimes having the best intentions can be detrimental to health, so we need to do activities that don't compromise our health negatively.
2. Making time to do things that nurture you is important in the work/life/caring balance. A recent article reported that mindfulness, yoga, prayer, exercise, talking therapies and maintaining hobbies/interests can help reduce distress for carers (Lebert et al. 2015).

Getting Your Life in Balance

Step 1 of the first cornerstone of caring is to review the work/life balance of both the carer and service user. When life is balanced too far on one side, this can disturb the equilibrium, which in turn can affect caring for yourself and others. A good way to address this issue is to plan time more effectively: what are your priorities, aims and goals? Think about these and then you can plan accordingly where this fits in your life. Activity scheduling is a great way of creating a physical plan to address the work/life balance; we include examples in Tables 7.1–7.3 of how this can be done. After evaluating these schedules, both the carer and service user should attempt to complete their own activity schedules (blank copies for your use have been included in this chapter).

Table 7.1 An example of my completed activity schedule

Day/ Activity	Monday	Tuesday	Wednesday	Thursday	Friday	Saturday	Sunday
Morning	Work	Work	Work	Work	Work	Bootcamp	Lie-in
Afternoon	Study	Work	Study	Work	Work	Shopping	Relaxation
Evening	Cooking	Roller skating	Kickboxing	Cooking	Socialise	Relaxation	Socialise
Night	Watch TV/ sleep	Watch TV/ sleep	Watch TV/ sleep	Watch TV/ sleep	Party	Party	Sleep

Table 7.2 An example of a carer's completed activity schedule

Day/ Activity	Monday	Tuesday	Wednesday	Thursday	Friday	Saturday	Sunday
Morning	Work	Work	Work	Work	Work	Work	Yoga
Afternoon	Work	Work	Work	Cooking/ caring	Work	Socialise	Cooking/ caring
Evening	Cooking/ caring	Cooking/ caring	Cooking/ caring	Cooking/ caring	Relaxation	Watch TV	Family time
Night	Watch TV/ sleep	Watch TV/ sleep	Sleep	Sleep	Sleep	Sleep	Watch TV/ sleep

Table 7.3 An example of a service user's completed activity schedule

Day/ Activity	Monday	Tuesday	Wednesday	Thursday	Friday	Saturday	Sunday
Morning	Manage voices	Sleep	Volunteer	Lie-in	Sleep	Sleep	Sleep
Afternoon	Listen to music	Sleep	Sleep	See member of care team	Sleep	Sleep	Sleep
Evening	Watch TV	Manage voices	Listen to music	Exercise	Socialise	Socialise	Watch TV
Night	Sleep	Watch TV	Manage voices	Sleep	Watch TV	Sleep	Sleep

What is your opinion of these activity schedules? Are they balanced? What could be improved? What do you think the emotional situation in the household will be like? Please use the following space for comments.

_____

_____

_____

_____

_____

Tables 7.4 and 7.5 provide blank activity schedules for both the service user and carer to complete.

Name:
My activity schedule

Day/ Activity	Monday	Tuesday	Wednesday	Thursday	Friday	Saturday	Sunday
Morning							
Afternoon							
Evening							
Night							

Name:
My activity schedule

Day/ Activity	Monday	Tuesday	Wednesday	Thursday	Friday	Saturday	Sunday
Morning							
Afternoon							
Evening							
Night							

Once you have both completed your activity schedules, why not swap with each other and have a conversation about the balance of the schedule? What is the outcome from this? Does anything need to change? Is there enough time for meeting goals, socialising, relaxation and work? It is important that once you have created a schedule you are happy with, you are not driven by it and allow for some flexibility to avoid stress.

Flow activities are those that you participate in, in an almost a trance-like state; you are truly focused and anything else happening around you is not at the forefront of your attention. It is often found that the activities that you enjoy the most are 'flow' activities, as they are generally rewarding. The difference between doing a flow activity and doing a general activity is that flow activities require more physical or mental effort when first starting out and the reward, which is usually more pleasurable, is gained from doing the activity, more so than the end outcome. Art is an excellent example of a flow activity, as you often find yourself immersed within a zone with a clear set of goals and aims in sight.

To optimise the caring milieu, you should aim to encourage activities of flow within your lifestyle and the person you care for and not give up on hope.

Improving the Emotional Tone at Home

What is the emotional tone in your household? We should be aiming for an emotionally neutral tone when communicating. An emotionally neutral tone is not angry, anxious or overly involved. When communicating, the key is to always be curious, attentive and show interest in what the person you are caring for is saying to you. A good approach is to show an appropriate level of encouragement with a slightly distanced attitude. Mondal and Mishra (2015) report that many studies have found links between high expressed emotion within families and increase in relapse risk.

The theory behind emotional neutrality is that if we can leave our own emotions out of situations, then we can think more clearly about the interactions that we make with others and communication can become much improved.

Tips for Emotional Neutrality

- Be curious.
- Avoid expressing too much anxiety.
- Be encouraging without becoming pushy.
- Show interest and be attentive.
- Be respectful of other views.

Columbo is a great fictional TV example of somebody demonstrating good emotional neutrality when talking with others. Columbo stays calm and asks questions in a curious and interested manner.

Examples of a Counterproductive Emotional Tone

Example 1: Joan is a carer for her daughter, Leanne, who has psychosis; she tries her best to encourage Leanne to get involved in activities. The more Joan tries to encourage, the more Leanne withdraws socially and the more time she spends in her room sleeping. Leanne views this encouragement as criticism and becomes increasingly distressed.

Example 2: Andy wants to help his brother, Chris, to recover as quickly as possible; to do this, he tries to help in every aspect of Chris's life by doing everything for him. This kindness displayed similarly leads to Chris disengaging from Andy and others, among other negative symptoms.

Questions

What is going wrong in these situations?

What can a carer/friend do?

The problem with these scenarios is that the emotional tone is unhelpful because it is not emotionally neutral. As a carer/friend we can try to help by practicing the earlier tips for emotional neutrality within the household. Another important factor in achieving emotional neutrality is recognising and respecting the symptoms of psychosis.

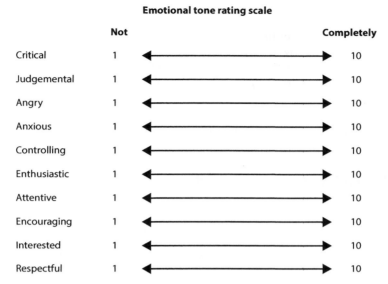

Figure 7.1 Emotional tone rating scale

Table 7.6 Examples of balancing the emotional tone.

Example	How to balance the emotional tone
'Why don't you get a grip?'	'This must be very difficult. Would you like to talk about it? I'd like to understand the situation more'
'You just need to get a job and then everything will be okay'	'Have you considered looking for work? It may be helpful. If you want, I can help'
'I don't have time for your nonsense. What you're saying isn't true'	'You have some interesting thoughts. How have you come to these conclusions?'

Have an up-front discussion with your carer/person you are caring for about your current interaction with each other and how it could be improved. What works well, what doesn't work and how does this make you feel? For example, the person you are caring for may find that the emotional tone within the household is too critical. Figure 7.1 provides a scale for you both to complete; once complete, swap the scales with each other and discuss. Discussion of all dimensions may be too much, so perhaps at first just focus on one dimension, such as the criticalness of conversation.

After practicing ameliorating the emotional tone, revisit the scale and repeat to see what else can be done.

Examples of rephrasing your language to balance the emotional tone are presented in Table 7.6.

Activating Self-Nurturing

Self-nurturing is vital to one's ability to cope. For some people, this can be switched off due to difficult life circumstances, but there is good news: it can be reactivated! Deactivation can occur due to many reasons such as trauma, bullying and neglect.

Compassionate Writing

Compassionate writing can be a great way of reactivating self-nurturing. Paul Gilbert (2007) describes this nicely in his work about writing a compassionate letter. A compassionate letter is an emotional piece of writing based on your feelings and the feelings of your compassionate self. Your compassionate self is the caring, understanding and nurturing side of yourself.

The main focus of compassionate letter writing should be your feelings based on being empathetic, respectful, reflective, supportive and positive.

Sample of a Compassionate Letter

Dear Thomas,

I am sorry to see you so distressed recently; you've felt guilty about your situation at work, your current lifestyle and your relationship with others. It is understandable that if there are too many demands in your life that you will feel strained. You've juggled work demands, meaning it has been difficult to look after yourself well.

Not prioritising your own needs has made you feel miserable, and you miss the closeness of the relationships with your loved ones. It seems as if you deserve a break. Remember when you felt stressed a few years ago, you coped well and were able to overcome these difficulties. You can do this!

Love from,

My compassionate self

Task: Both carer and service user should write a compassionate letter to themselves. After writing your letters, re-read them. Are they critical or judgemental? Are you negative towards yourself? Writing a compassionate letter can take some time, and you may find yourself writing this letter a few times before it becomes truly compassionate.

Letter writing isn't the only way of activating self-nurturing; there are other compassion-based techniques, such as creating a fantasy identity of your ideal self that you can create a mental image of or even loving and kindness meditation.

Imagery

Creating a compassionate self-image is a very individualistic process, as it is based on your ideals. It can be a powerful tool in self-care, as it encourages you to nurture yourself in a more loving way. I would like my compassionate self to be the person described in Figure 7.2. This person is a strong, young female who radiates energy and is able to find positives in any situation. Why not try creating a compassionate self-image? When doing this, please bear in mind that your compassionate self wants what's best for you but does not tell you what to do or criticise you; they are there to be supportive of you and encourage growth.

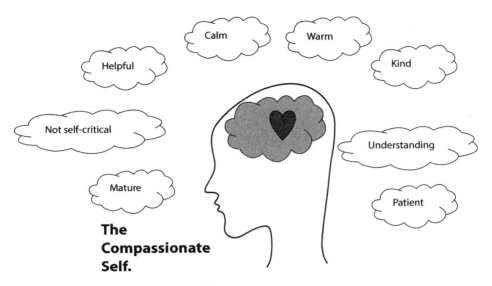

Figure 7.2 A positive and compassionate self-image

Questions

What is your compassionate self like?

What qualities does your compassionate self possess?

How would they use these qualities to help you in your experiences?

Loving and Kindness Meditation

You can practice activating loving and kindness in a number of ways. Why not try chanting to yourself positive, inspirational quotes or words which invoke feelings of love and kindness? For example, 'Fill me with love and let happiness in'. Similar to using compassionate imagery, you can also spend time picturing a happy you. What does this person look like? What are they doing? Positively reflecting on the encouraging qualities that you possess can also form part of your meditation routine. The techniques described can be used to activate loving and kindness for yourself or perhaps another close relationship where you feel that your compassion towards them may be somewhat lacking. In the latter case the technique is alike, but the imagery, verbal chanting and reflection are focused towards that other person; for example, you may say, 'Fill them with happiness and peace', or you may reflect on the kind acts that they have done in their lives. It is important that if you choose to use this technique you first work on activating your own self-compassion through meditation and then your compassion towards others. This type of meditation can be practiced in short pulses throughout the day. Research shows that there are many benefits to adopting this type of meditation, such as improvement in negative symptoms of psychosis and helping carers to cope better (Hoffman et al. 2011; Johnson et al. 2009).

Communicating

Communication can get stuck in a rut for many reasons, and people often become comfortable with a particular communication style. It can be quite difficult to recognise this, as we tend to be more naturally able to find faults in others than in ourselves. When communicating we can often be listening to another person but not actually be fully immersed in that conversation. This can happen due to your mind wandering, checking text messages or perhaps over-focussing on how you feel in relation to what the other person is saying. Even sometimes I can find myself already thinking of what I want to communicate without considering or allowing the other person to finish what they have said. By engaging in these bad habits, we miss a vital step in the communication process: listening.

The key to *real* listening is active listening; this involves being proactive to show the speaker that you are actively engaged. This can be demonstrated by nodding, maintaining eye contact, displaying congruent expressions and using verbal cues in conversation (e.g. yes, um, okay).

Body language is also a vital component of the five pillars; it can make the difference in how open somebody is to communicating. Your body needs to be open and congruent with the speech that accompanies it. Be aware of the body language of the person you are talking with also.

When somebody is speaking with you, reflecting and paraphrasing what one has said can help you to summarise and confirm the information provided. It also offers you the opportunity to clarify the main points of the conversation.

Most importantly, don't forget your humour; life isn't always about seriousness, so enjoy it! Using humour appropriately can take the tension out of those difficult conversations.

Befriending

Befriending is a technique that has been popular with carers, maybe due to the discussion and embrace of shared experiences. Befriending differs from general social interaction in the fact that it is more structured and goal focused. A slot to befriend should be made once a week for a 30-minute period – more than this may be too demanding for yourself and the person you are caring for. Befriending has been shown to be effective in aiding improvement in psychotic symptoms and is even comparable to CBT in the short term (Sensky et al. 2000). Befriending is not CBT; there is no active formulation of life events involved. Also it requires no active use of CBT techniques or teaching the techniques to others.

When starting this befriending conversation, it is important that the focus is on neutral topics which don't evoke extreme reactions and that these topics are non-threatening for either party. If such topics arise, it is important that you are non-confrontational in your approach or response. Sometimes during this session ideas or beliefs that may seem unusual arise from the person whom you are befriending; it is highly important in this situation that you do not collude with these ideas. For instance, if the person you are caring for decides that members of their family have been possessed by aliens, being non-collusive would involve acknowledging what they have said but also gently replying in an emotionally neutral manner that from your experience the family members have acted strangely in the past (if this is true), but you haven't noticed anything out of the ordinary which would make you think that they could be aliens. The next step would be to move the conversation to a more neutral topic such as good Christmas experiences that you have both shared with the family. An example of being collusive would be to agree with the person that family members are aliens.

The aim of a befriending session should be to reduce distress; therefore, you should be empathetic in your approach and response and supportive and accepting of the situation. Topics during this period should be focused on the past, which activates positive shared memories. Setting a regular slot to do this may be a useful aid in improving the caring milieu and can be a fun and enjoyable experience for you both.

Hope

The introduction of hope and recovery should be a strong theme that encompasses all of the five pillars. The fact that you're reading this book tells me that hope is not lost and optimism exists. Optimism is key to effective caring and can help instil optimism in others.

Summary of Key Coping Techniques: Dos and Don'ts

Do ... Optimise your work/life/caring balance

Do ... Activate self-nurturing

Do ... Take steps to improve your emotional tone

Do ... Make effective use of communication

Do ... Introduce hope and flow activities

Don't ... Be overly critical of yourself or the person you may be caring for

Don't ... Let communication get stuck in a rut

Don't ... Lose hope

Acknowledgements

Maggie Douglas-Bailey helped to develop the flow and compassion sections in this chapter.

References

Gilbert, P. (2007) Compassionate letter writing: Therapist notes. Retrieved 5 April 2016 from www.compassionatemind.co.uk/resources/Compassionate_Letter_Writing.pdf.

Hoffman, S. P., Grossman, G. & Hinton, D. E. (2011) Loving-kindness and compassion meditation: Potential for psychological interventions. *Clinical Psychology Review*, 31(7), 1126–32.

Johnson, D. P., Penn, D. L., Fredrickson, B. L., Meyer, P. S., Kring, A. M. & Brantley, M. (2009) Loving-kindness meditation to enhance recovery from negative symptoms of schizophrenia. *Journal of Clinical Psychology*, 65, 499–509.

Lebert L., Spencer, H. & Turkington, D. (2015) Caring for relatives with schizophrenia: A role for stress reduction and CBT techniques training. *The British Journal of Psychiatry*. Retrieved 5 April 2016 from http://bjp.rcpsych.org/content/caring-relatives-schizophrenia-role-stress-reduction-and-cbt-techniques-training

Mondal, A., & Mishra, D. (2015). Expressed emotion and coping strategies in the caregivers of schizophrenia patients. *Journal of Contemporary Psychological Research*, 2(2), 1–7.

Sensky, T., Turkington, D., Kingdon, D., et al. (2000) A randomized controlled trial of cognitive–behavioural therapy for persistent symptoms in schizophrenia resistant to medication. *Archives of General Psychiatry,* 57, 165–72.

Further Reading

Compassionate Letter Writing

Gilbert, P. (2007) Compassionate letter writing: Therapist notes. Retrieved 5 April 2016 from www.compassionatemind.co.uk/resources/Compassionate_Letter_Writing.pdf.

Compassion-Focused Exercises

Gilbert, P. (2010) Training our minds in, with and for compassion: An introduction to concepts and compassion-focused exercises. Retrieved 5 April 2016 from www.compassionatemind.co.uk/downloads/training_materials/3.%20Clinical_patient_handout.pdf.

Meditation

Kornfield, J. (2008) *The art of forgiveness, lovingkindness, and peace.* New York: Bantam Dell.

Links to Other Chapters

- Chapter 13, improving self-care, attention, motivation and social functioning
- Chapter 8, effective coping: Carer and service user self-care
- Chapter 12, compassion-focused approaches for clients, families and health care providers

Effective Coping
Carer and Service User Self-Care

Latoyah Lebert

Key Points

1. Identify if there is a problem that you need to cope with.
2. Usually the first attempts to cope don't work and we need to experiment with new ones.
3. It is really useful to ask others to help us cope better.
4. Coping is built on a normalising explanation.
5. We need to find ways to cope with emotions as well as symptoms like hallucinations or paranoia.
6. It is often useful to begin with distraction and then move to focusing in order to extract more meaning from the experience.

Introduction

Effective coping styles are crucial for success in life. Everybody faces adversity in life, but it is how we react to these situations that often dictates future happiness and current levels of distress. This chapter provides both service user and carer with some tools to be able to cope with the distress associated with having upsetting emotions (anger, sadness, guilt, shame, anxiety and boredom) and also psychotic experiences (in particular, voices and paranoia). It is, of course, often the situation that if we can cope better with the emotions, then the psychotic experiences will become less distressing.

Personal Disclosure

When reflecting back on how I have coped in adverse situations, there are definitely times where I can say that my strategies were ineffective to say the least!

I visited Amsterdam last year with a friend and happened to wander into a coffee shop for a snack. I ordered a chocolate cake and a couple of hours later began to feel strange. Everything looked distorted and I thought everybody knew that I was stoned in the middle of Anne Frank's house. I felt scared, as if everybody was talking about me and felt as if crowds of fuzzy people were walking towards me. To cope with this situation I had to sit down in order to feel the ground under me and try to make sense of what was going on around me. I was able to work out a normalising explanation: I wasn't 'going mad' I had inadvertently consumed a large amount of cannabis. I was now able to understand why the chocolate cake was so expensive! I told my friend what I was experiencing, and she decided that a good coping strategy would be to take me to a restaurant for lots of food. When the food arrived I felt as if everybody was watching me and that my arms had extended so much I could not hold my knife and fork, so was forced to give up on eating. My friend then decided that the restaurant was not a good idea and walked me back to the hostel. I used a variety of coping strategies back at the hostel such as drinking lots of water and sitting in the common area talking with strangers about my experience.

What Were the Positive Aspects of Coping?

So the most important aspects of coping here were the ability to have a normalising explanation, grounding and basic reality testing. It was important to be able to ask for coping assistance and to have a friend around and then try different approaches until something worked.

Another Personal Disclosure

Another experience I had was in Jerusalem at a conference. I had decided to go on a city tour with a senior colleague, which started off well. Unfortunately he lost my phone in a city centre café but I had not realised this until we were miles away at the Mount of Olives. Once I realised it was not in his possession, I became panicky and angry. I didn't really think through what I was doing and acted almost automatically. I walked 10 paces ahead of him and ignored the senior colleague and stormed all the way back to where I thought my phone could possibly be. But we both got lost. This made me even angrier with him and the situation. I was not coping well with my anger and felt even more stressed. Finally we reached the café, and a worker came up to the senior colleague and asked him if he had lost a phone. I immediately felt an overwhelming sense of relief, but the senior colleague was feeling so guilty that he gave away all of the money we had with us (£50) to the worker as a reward. This meant that we had no money for a taxi and had to walk several miles back to the conference.

How Might We Have Coped Differently in This Situation?

I clearly didn't cope well with the emotion of anger. What would you have done? One possible plan might have been for me to take a few deep breaths and consider that phones are often lost. The senior colleague didn't purposely lose my phone and had actually made a kind gesture to carry it for me. To find this phone I needed to cope with my anger so that we could navigate our way back to the café without getting lost.

The senior colleague didn't cope at all well with the emotion of guilt. What would you have done? He did try to apologise, but I refused to listen to him and kept storming ahead. He needed to realise that he was feeling excessively guilty and needed to speak to me again to negotiate a sensible reward (maybe £20?).

This shows that all of us every day need to make coping decisions not only about emotions but also about the symptoms that we suffer from. Coping can always be improved upon. It is a work in progress.

Experiences of Famous People

J. K. Rowling, a famous author known for the hugely popular Harry Potter novels, was rejected by publishers several times before reaching success. This process of repeated rejection along with adverse life events led to a deep depression. Rowling coped with rejection and failure by accepting that she may never succeed and focusing on her passion that was writing and setting herself small, achievable goals.

Gandhi, a nonviolent protester from India, coped with numerous assassination attempts and arrests by keeping his main goal for an independent, tolerant and fair society at the forefront of his mind. He used the search for truth to overcome difficulties – this was a great coping strategy as it allowed him to remain focused and not engage in violent protests. Here Gandhi's passion was social and political in nature rather than the creative nature that Rowling's passion followed.

Do you have a passion that you are able to focus on?

So What Can We Conclude?

Having a positive mind-set and having a goal to aim for can act as a motivational tool. Expressing your feelings and letting others know what you are experiencing can be helpful in coping. Acknowledging your emotions and being able to recognise whether you are reacting to the emotion in an effective way is important.

What Are the Problems that You Are Currently Coping With? What Techniques Do You or the Person Who You Care for Use to Deal with Symptoms of Psychosis?

Think about the techniques that you use to cope: Are they effective? List them in Table 8.1.

Have a discussion with your carer/loved one about how these strategies help or hinder you. If you are unsure whether they are helpful or not, you can try measuring symptom distress using a scale from 1 to 10 to measure symptoms/experiences over a period of a week whilst using the previously listed coping strategies. If the strategies prove ineffective, try some of the other simple techniques that we discuss next in this chapter.

Examples of Effective Coping Strategies that Are Less Complex

> Example 1: John is a 49-year-old male who enjoyed rock concerts, writing and listening to music; he used to regularly write lyrics and had a songbook collection. Since developing psychosis John has now given up all of his previous interests. He frequently hears voices, which are critical and distracting. The voices often tell John that he is a bad person who

Table 8.1 Identifying your current coping strategies

What is the problem?	How do I cope?
1. The army are spying on me...	Close all the curtains and blinds
2.	
3.	
4.	
5.	
6.	
7.	
8.	
9.	
10.	

deserves punishment. To cope with these voices, John often self-harms and responds by talking aloud back to the voices. This results in scars on John's body, which he tries to disguise due to feeling embarrassed; it also results in low self-esteem. The combination of distress, low self-esteem and embarrassment will inevitably worsen the voices – the coping strategies simply haven't worked.

What Simple Techniques May Help John in This Situation?

Learning an Instrument

Learning an instrument is an excellent technique, as it focuses your attention on the here and now. The melodies of an instrument can be relaxing, and it requires concentration to learn a new skill. Once this skill has been learnt, you may try playing with others or joining a band; this can lead to increased social contact, which facilitates successful coping.

Subvocalisation

Reading aloud is a simple but effective technique which can help with coping with voices and delusions, as your mental efforts are going into absorbing and vocalising the content of the book. The concept of this idea is that reading aloud overpowers intrusive thoughts or voices, as it disrupts 'inner speech'. John may find that using this technique helps with the frequency of voices and the associated distress.

Graphotherapy

Graphotherapy has a considerable evidence base in the literature as an effective tool for those with severe mental health problems. The sheer process of writing down internal events is impactful. Using this approach, the service user writes a page every day to record what the voices have been saying. It soon becomes apparent that the content is both negative and repetitive. John tried this technique, and after two weeks of working on this task, he threw his diary down and announced to his therapist that the voices were 'boring, same old rubbish every day'. From this point onwards, he felt more empowered to get on with his usual activities and became less involved and frightened by selectively listening to the voices' content.

Examples of Effective Coping Strategies that Are Slightly More Complex

Example 2: Charles is a 28-year-old male who was a sci-fi fanatic and regularly attended comic conventions and played video games until his symptoms began. Charles now hears the voice of an alien – the voice says that Charles is the chosen one to work for them in their mission to take over the planet. Charles believes this to be true, as he believes the voices began when a wasp stung him in his ear on his 17th birthday. He thought this sting gave him a special ability, allowing the aliens to communicate with him. Charles is distressed that the aliens are coming and have chosen him to communicate with, so he regularly directs this anger towards his family by shouting at them. This anger is exacerbated due to the fact that his family do not believe him. Charles has been to the police station on several occasions, asking to be detained in order to have more protection from the aliens. Charles is experiencing a range of emotions here, from anger to fear, but the techniques that he has employed such as expressing anger and visiting the police have made his beliefs stronger.

What Slightly More Complex Techniques May Help Charles in This Situation?

Attentional Training

People living with psychosis are often tuned into their voices and beliefs – in other words they are hyper-alert to what the voices are doing. To disrupt the cognitive attentional state which serves to maintain troublesome voices, the service user is trained to practice shifting his or her attention to different auditory stimuli (for example, the ticking of a clock, the sound of traffic, radio or birdsong). Repeated practice of attentional shifts may lead to an increase in confidence, in terms of being able to move attention away from the voices and thoughts to promote a less emotionally engaged coping style. A training recording is available from www.mct-institute.com.

Rational Responding

All voices contain distortions, as do most automatic thoughts. The first step is to write the voice content down on a white board. This is a focusing breakthrough, as the voices are exposed, usually for the first time, to independent scientific analysis. Each voice can be examined individually to look for a level of veracity. Has the voice got it right? Or is there evidence of distortion such as magnification, labelling, mind-reading error or selective abstraction? On generating a rational response, the service user can speak back to the voice. This is done gently and quietly to 'correct' the distortion in terms of what the voice is saying. These distortions are repeatedly identified, and a more rational statement is fed back to the voice, for example, Voice: 'He is a loser, no-one cares about him'. Rational response: 'I am a human being, sometimes I win and sometimes I lose and I do have a girlfriend who cares about me'. The rational response can then be written on a card or recorded on a tape or mobile phone to remind the service user of the rational responses outwith the therapy session.

Voice Postponement

Similar to coping with worry, you can postpone voices by confining them to have their say at a period specified by the service user. For example, Charles may make the conscious decision to postpone responding to the voice of an alien until 7 p.m. He may even put a limit on the time that he allows the voice to talk; for example, a 15-minute time cap may be put in place. This strategy will allow Charles to begin to resume day-to-day activities and to take control of the auditory hallucinations that he experiences. Learning a new habit does not always result in instant escape from voices, and it can take many repetitions of a behaviour before it becomes a habit; therefore, you shouldn't give up at the first hurdle.

Other Techniques

Music

Listening to melodic, meaningful music can be a useful distraction technique from voices and paranoid beliefs, as it focuses your attention elsewhere. Music should be listened to aloud through a player rather than headphones, as wearing headphones can increase isolation. What is meaningful can be very individualistic; you should explore listening to different types of sounds and note how you feel afterwards.

Mindfulness

Practising mindfulness such as mindful walking, breathing and eating can help reduce one's sense of distress. However, in cases where you have experienced some kind of trauma or have the tendency to dissociate, mindfulness can be unhelpful (Turkington, Lebert & Spencer, 2016). For example, where the person hears the voice of the abuser, using a focusing technique such as mindfulness may increase negative emotions without appropriate professional psychological support.

Animals

Some studies have found that spending time with animals has positive benefits for psychological wellbeing. Kanat-Maymona, Antebia and Zilcha-Manob (2016) suggested that people who have pets have higher levels of self-value.

Nature

A review of nature-based therapies such as rambling, hill walking, birdwatching, etc. has found that they can be beneficial in terms of symptom reduction for a number of health conditions, including schizophrenia (Annerstedt & Wåhborg, 2011).

After reading this chapter you should have some idea of what coping techniques are efficient and what you would like to try. Table 8.2 provides spaces for you to record your ideas.

My main coping techniques to deal with my problems that I now plan to try out are ...

Measurement

Individual coping techniques that are chosen by the service user should be practiced each day and scored on a 10-point scale to measure efficacy in terms of reducing the frequency and distress associated with the psychotic experience. After seven days the first coping style can be reviewed and either extended for a further 7 days or swapped to a different coping technique if there is no evidence of clinical improvement.

Table 8.2 New coping strategies which I will try to use

What is the problem?	How will I cope?
1. The army are spying on me...	Tell my loved ones about the situation
2.	
3.	
4.	
5.	
6.	
7.	
8.	
9.	
10.	

Keeping a record of how you are doing when using these techniques may be useful in aiding you in your discovery of activities that help you to cope. What is the most helpful? What is the least helpful?

Table 8.3 provides a chart so that you can record these experiences.

Looking at the completed table, is there anything that you will do differently to cope?

Table 8.3 Measuring the benefits of a coping strategy

Coping technique	What were my thoughts whilst doing this?	How did I feel whilst doing this? 0 = not at all 10 = extremely	Severity of voices/ paranoid thoughts 0 = none at all 10 = worst ever experienced
Example: Listening to electronic repetitive music with no vocals	Boring	Happy = 0 Relaxed = 0 Distressed = 5	8 (really bad voices)
		Happy = Relaxed = Distressed =	
		Happy = Relaxed = Distressed =	
		Happy = Relaxed = Distressed =	
		Happy = Relaxed = Distressed =	
		Happy = Relaxed = Distressed =	
		Happy = Relaxed = Distressed =	
		Happy = Relaxed = Distressed =	
		Happy = Relaxed = Distressed =	
		Happy = Relaxed = Distressed =	
		Happy = Relaxed = Distressed =	

Summary of Key Coping Techniques: Dos and Don'ts

Do ... talk to close family or friends about your experiences and coping techniques.

Do ... work on a trial-and-error basis when seeking an appropriate coping technique.

Do ... start with the simpler techniques.

Don't ... persevere if your symptoms get worse.

Don't ... give up without practising.

References

Annerstedt, M., & Wähborg, P. (2011) Nature-assisted therapy: Systematic review of controlled and observational studies. *Scandinavian Journal of Public Health*, 39, 371–88.

Kanat-Maymona, Y., Antebia, A. & Zilcha-Manob, S. (2016) Basic psychological need fulfillment in human–pet relationships and well-being. *Personality and Individual Differences*, 92, 69–73.

Turkington, D., Lebert, L.N., & Spencer, H.M. (2016) Auditory hallucinations in schizophrenia: Helping service users to develop effective coping strategies. *British Journal of Psychiatry Advances*. 22 (6), 391–6

Further Reading

Wells, A. (2011) *Metacognitive therapy for anxiety and depression*. New York: Guilford.

Websites/Other Info

Metacognitive information: www.mct-institute.com.

Links to Other Chapters

- Chapter 6
- Chapter 7

Caring about Delusions and Unusual Beliefs

Douglas Turkington

Key Points

1. Use a befriending style and try to remain emotionally neutral.
2. Ask curious questions.
3. Remember there will be a seed of truth in the new belief.
4. Help your relative or friend to consider other possible explanations.
5. Do homework exercises with the person to discover new information.
6. Keep in touch with the psychiatric team or primary care physician.
7. Raise any red flag situations immediately with the psychiatric team.

Introduction

Unusual beliefs are formed at various times by almost everyone in society. Good examples might include falling in love, religious conversion and affiliation with certain groups such as bikers, punks and goths. In schizophrenia and the psychotic disorders, new unusual beliefs are given the name *delusions*, in that they are perceived to be held in the face of evidence to the contrary or to be bizarre in nature and to be beliefs that other people from their society, culture and background simply cannot agree with. Delusions are hallmark symptoms of schizophrenia and can be extremely distressing and disabling. Delusions, however, are often responsive to change with CBT. This chapter outlines what carers, friends and service users themselves can do by using the most basic befriending and CBT techniques to help the psychiatric treatment team reduce the distress and disability of these new beliefs.

Personal Disclosure

At the age of 15 years I fell in love and my behaviour completely changed! I stopped seeing my friends, stopped playing football, became dreamy and preoccupied, seemed unable to put the phone down and centred my whole life around this new person who I had only just met. My girlfriend ended things six weeks later (she then formed a new relationship with an older boy). This experience was hugely painful, but my delusion of being in love did gradually change and eventually resolved completely. At 18 years of age I fairly suddenly formed the belief that I was a Christian, and again my behaviour and moods changed profoundly. This belief seemed to relate to a search for meaning in life during late adolescence and proved to be longer lasting.

These are just two examples from my personal experience of dramatic belief change. Neither of these beliefs would have been seen as bizarre by others in my society. However, if I had undertaken these belief changes in a different culture (e.g. as an orthodox Jew or in communist China), both belief changes would have been questioned as the possible emergence of mental illness. Certainly falling in love in such cultures would be expected to occur following a period of family negotiation about suitability. A Christian conversion in either of the cultures mentioned would be seen as non–culture-syntonic and possibly a symptom of mental disorder.

So What Can We Conclude?

1. The human mind is set up to make sudden changes of belief, and these changes then shift the person's mood and behaviour.
2. Such belief changes are related to the person's culture. For example, in our Western society where the Internet and social media are very much imbedded in our culture, people form suspicious or paranoid beliefs about being watched and about others following them or trying to gather information about them. Whereas in China, suspicious or paranoid beliefs might relate to spitting or courtship rituals. Spitting in public and ritualised courtship are accepted aspects of Chinese culture.
3. Belief changes, when made, are often resistant to change, but they can start to shift and become more flexible, particularly with the use of certain CBT techniques such as a review of the evidence and reality testing.
4. A newly formed belief is often resistant to change, particularly if confronted.
5. A new belief may become the dominant driver of emotion and behaviour, but alternative beliefs are still there and can be brought into discussion.

Positive Aspects of New Belief Formation

There is a link between schizophrenia, which can involve the formation of new beliefs that others view as surprising, and examples of breakthroughs in creativity both in the sciences and in the arts. For example, Albert Einstein stated that he himself was no genius and that his mind presented the theory of relativity and other massive scientific breakthroughs to him in a fully formed state. Sudden jumps in knowledge can therefore come from a creative (seemingly psychotic) area of the mind. Interestingly, Albert Einstein had a son who spent most of his life in asylum care with chronic schizophrenia. Another example of this is John Nash (a mathematics professor) as portrayed in the film *A Beautiful Mind* who said that his delusional beliefs came exactly from the same place in his mind as his mathematical genius. The author, J.K. Rowling, of the hugely successful Harry Potter series indicated that she dreamed all the plots and simply had to write them down. Carl Gustav Jung, perhaps the most creative psychiatrist of his age, had a number of psychotic experiences throughout his life and yet made highly impressive breakthroughs in relation to the psychology and psychiatric management of the psychotic disorders and the individual development of the mind. The capacity to have creative thoughts and to form new beliefs, therefore, is one that has been extremely important for the advancement of the human race.

An Example of a New Belief

Josh is an 18-year-old man who was devastated following a failed relationship. He was then the victim of bullying and started abusing cannabis. At that time he formed a new belief that the Mexican mafia were watching his house and intended to kill him if he left the premises. He stayed indoors, becoming increasingly isolated.

Questions

Why has this new paranoid belief emerged?

What can a carer/friend do?

This new belief is on a spectrum with normal beliefs. At this age Josh is prone to forming new beliefs, particularly around the key age of relationship formation and breakdown.

A study by Samarasekara and colleagues (2007) showed that for very paranoid people, befriending was a helpful way of reducing the person's paranoid thinking. The befriending approach is designed to gradually increase social contact by discussing topics that are not too deep or emotional. If the service user asks the befriender if they believe that their new (delusional) belief(s) are true, then the befriender would simply say that they did not know much about that subject but the befriender would acknowledge that there could be some truth in it, as they themselves had encountered suspicious thoughts in the past. For example, the befriender might say to the service user 'do you remember that time we thought there was a man spying on us with binoculars? But it turned out that he was a birdwatcher!' The befriender would then steer the discussion back on to the person's previous hobbies, interests, friendships, etc., in an attempt to distract the service user from the preoccupation associated with their delusions. A carer, in the face of a strong paranoid belief, might initially use this type of befriending. Then it is possible to ask a few CBT questions about the nature of the new belief in a gentle and inquisitive way.

For example:

How does Josh know that the Mexican mafia are involved?

Could there be any other possible explanations?

How could we test some of these other explanations out?

Can Josh think of some other possible explanations to make sense of what is going on?

Well, if it is the mafia then how do we know that it is not the Russians rather than the Mexican mafia? Or could it be something to do with the bullying that previously happened? Or could it be that he has been very upset, taking things too painfully, not sleeping well or smoking cannabis which has fuelled some of these suspicious thoughts and led to a new belief?

In this way a carer or family friend might move from a befriending stance to a questioning approach to find out more about the new belief and help generate some other possibilities to explain what is happening. This needs to be done slowly and sensitively. Closed-ended questions should not be used and new explanations not put forward as a means to try and convince the person that they are wrong.

It would be reasonable for a carer to say something close to the original belief, for example, I did not know the Mexican mafia were active in this area – where could I find out more about this? This is useful because it allows the carer to do some homework, for example, looking in the local newspapers with Josh to look for information in relation to the Mexican mafia. This in turn could help him re-evaluate his belief when he is guided to the realisation that there are no reports of the Mexican mafia in the area.

New beliefs can be invested in strong emotions such as fear, anger or sadness. Useful carer-based CBT approaches are listed in Table 9.1 to help reduce the intensity of these feelings, which, while not only distressing, are also linked to safety behaviours (e.g. staying indoors for prolonged periods) which will worsen and maintain the new belief.

Table 9.1 Examples of feelings, behaviours and thoughts linked to new beliefs: thinking and acting differently

Feelings linked to new belief	Behaviour	Thoughts	Alternative ways of thinking	Possible actions
Fear	Pale, restless, sweaty, fast speech, heart palpitations	I'm going to be in danger and I can't cope.	I'm OK just now. There are things that I can do to cope.	Relaxation training, mindful breathing, walking, yoga, distraction exercises
Anger	Raised voice, clenched fists, staring	It's not fair, something must be done.	I can't demand fairness. I don't know who they might be. I need more information.	Distraction using hobbies; imagery exercises
Sadness	Sad expression, reduced speech, tearfulness, poor appetite, weight loss	I'm a bad person. The situation is hopeless, and the future is not worthwhile.	I'm a human being and basically as good as anybody else. The world contains good and bad things and the future might be OK.	Keep a diary of simple activities and score these activities on a scale of 0 to 10 in terms of achievement and enjoyment

In the presence of extreme sadness, carers and friends should always ask the service user directly if they have any thoughts or plans to harm themselves or commit suicide. If they do elicit these type of responses, the carer or friend should stay with the person, make the situation safe and then phone the case manager and emergency services. This is a red flag situation – always ask.

A More Complex Example

The following example demonstrates a situation in which the belief does not seem to follow on from the events beforehand but seems to cover up feelings linked to previous events.

Tom, aged 52 years, had a long criminal record for theft, and after having seen a purple light in his prison cell, he came to believe that he was the second coming of Jesus Christ. He reported being plagued by a recurring image of a lady screaming (his victim) when he had attempted to steal her handbag. Here the new belief has arisen to cover unbearable feelings of guilt for his crime(s). With the new belief that he is Jesus Christ, Tom believed he had the power to wipe away his own sin and guilt and that of others. This kind of new belief is difficult for a carer or friend to cope with, as Tom was spending a lot of time preaching and inviting people to become his disciples.

Again in the face of a strongly held new belief we begin with a befriending approach. It is really important to talk to the service user. New beliefs can appear overpowering, but in fact they are quite fragile and will change over time if the correct approach is taken. Again we cannot collude or confront but we can ask questions within an emotionally neutral style. Examples might be: Tell me about the purple light; How does purple relate to Jesus? How did you feel before you saw the purple light? What events were taking place in your life before you started to believe that you were Jesus Christ?

It is usually the case that questioning a new belief in this way will start to reveal some underlying emotions. In this example, working with the person's guilt could be helpful. Let's find out more about the theft of the lady's handbag and any subsequent crimes. What was the motivation surrounding these crimes? If the guilt is so severe that Tom believes he deserves self-punishment, then how much punishment should he receive? Is it necessarily a life sentence?

A carer or friend can ask these helpful questions, as well as help uncover information about the new belief and attempt some social activities. Engaging the service user in social activities is important, as it works as a distraction technique to help guide the person away from becoming too preoccupied about their beliefs. However, on some occasions an expert therapist is needed. Signals for this are increasing distress, worsening self-care, the emergence of suicidal thoughts or self-harm or increasing anger. Call your case manager/psychiatrist or therapist. If in doubt, always call.

In Table 9.2, enter the key details of the new belief that you as a carer/service user are currently dealing with:

Table 9.2 My family member's new belief: a homework exercise

Belief	Feelings	Behaviour	Questions	Other alternative explanations	Possible actions

It can be really useful to consider examples of other service users who have developed new beliefs and moved on from them. Examples can be found in the Further Reading section.

Summary of Key CBT Techniques: Dos and Don'ts

Do ... be curious and ask open questions to find out more

Do ... stay friendly and neutral

Do ... ask about feelings

Do ... ask about any other possible explanations

Do ... offer to do homework to find out more

Do ... help by suggesting relaxing and interesting activities

Don't ... confront or collude with the new belief

Don't ... ask questions to disprove the new belief

Don't ... expect quick change

Reference

Samarasekara, N., Kingdon, D., Siddle, R., et al. (2007). Befriending patients with medication-resistant schizophrenia: Can psychotic symptoms predict treatment response? *Psychology and Psychotherapy*, 80(1), 97–106.

Further Reading

Freeman, D., Freeman, J. & Garety, P. (2006). *Overcoming paranoid & suspicious thoughts: A self-help guide using cognitive behavioural techniques*. London: Constable & Robinson Ltd.

Morrison, A., Renton, J., French, P. & Bentall, R. (2008). *Think you're crazy? Think again: A resource book for cognitive therapy for psychosis.* East Sussex: Routledge.

Turkington, D. et al. (2009). *Back to life, back to normality: Cognitive therapy, recovery and psychosis.* Cambridge: Cambridge University Press.

And on the following websites:

1. Paranoidthoughts.com
2. Psychosisresearch.com

Links to Other Chapters

It can be useful to look at worry and rumination (see Chapter 3) and also to undertake some compassionate mind exercises (see Chapter 12).

In relation to homework and looking for evidence, it might be useful to refer to Chapter 10 and Chapter 11.

My Story of Psychosis and CBT

David Couper, Latoyah Lebert

Key Points

1. Psychosis can be caused by a combination of events.
2. Victims of abuse are not to blame.
3. Having audio recordings of your therapy session is like having gold dust!
4. Changing your response to voices can help them to subside.
5. Perseverance with homework is the key to CBT success.

Introduction

This chapter takes you through the story of David's journey through psychosis, exploring his past traumas, experiences of psychosis and experiences with medication and therapy. David discusses both the successful and unsuccessful CBT techniques that he employed to deal with psychosis.

In the personal disclosure that follows David describes a harrowing account of his struggle with long term schizoaffective disorder. It was crucial that he develop trust with a CBT therapist in order that he could learn more about his frightening psychotic symptoms and learn how to work to reduce risk to self and others. He developed a 'staying alive plan' and learned to recognise triggers for risk to others. He was then able to explore his timeline and understand the roots of his psychosis. While doing so he worked on emotions of shame and anger which were exacerbating his symptoms. He learned how to question paranoid delusions, generate other explanations and test them out. He learned that voice hearing was common and generated coping strategies. He then started to gently correct the voices and declined to act on their commands. He achieved recovery, went back to work and married but remains aware of relapse triggers and how to respond to them.

Personal Disclosure

When I was around 21 years old, quite young and naïve, I heard nurses talking about me one day in the hospital; two of them were discussing my welfare and they said 'that David will not last until he's 30'. At that point I burst into tears and started banging my head on the wall. One of the nurses came in and she said, 'What's the matter David?' I just said, 'I need some diazepam', and that was the answer to everything in those days: medication. Some of those tablets knocked you out, and they would put you into your bed to forget about it. That's how it was in those days, and I felt destroyed. I felt 'there's no hope for me, there's no hope for me!'. Nobody had any hope for me in those days, not even my family. My family said, 'You are away, you are too far gone'. Well, I'm 49 now and I've conquered my mental illness. I have actually conquered it through CBT. My therapist was a miracle man, a miracle worker, and he is the reason I am alive here today.

I was working seven days a week, 14 to 16 hours per day, as a tailor and I was drinking a lot and having a happy life. I was really happy in my life – or at least I thought I was. I was drinking a lot because that is what you did in the 1980s and the 1990s, just going out watching the football match and drinking 19 pints during the day and 19 pints at night time. It was crazy, getting lock-in's when the landlord would 'close the pub' at 11pm but we all stayed in there drinking until the early hours of the morning. I really drank a lot in those days, but I was kinda unhappy. I used to cry a lot, and looking back in hindsight, it was because of the abuse I suffered in the past. I was suffering, and when I got drunk, I always used to cry my eyes out and suffer flashbacks and things like that. But the next day I got up for work 6 a.m., bright as a button, away to work again, happy as Larry! I used to have a big crowd around me, and I attracted a crowd because I had the 'gift of the gab' and everyone wanted to be in my company.

One time I got involved with these guys who I thought were nice guys. I was out one night with them and it was horrendous – it was like a horror movie. These guys gave me a pint of lager and made a bet with me that I couldn't drink it. I drank it. It was mixed with LSD, acid, cocaine and a combination of all sorts of drugs. I then sat down and started seeing brains and horrible pictures around me and I became disorientated. I then went into different pubs trying to drink lots of water and eventually I jumped into the river. Before jumping in the river my girlfriend tried to get me to go to bed, but I couldn't get to bed. I jumped through the upstairs window. I was chasing my brain out of the window – I could literally see the brain out of the window and plants moving. I felt like I was in a film in the sky where I was naked and I was conscious of it happening. In reality, I was running through the Quayside in my underpants covered in cuts on my feet and hands and then I jumped in the river. Along came a policeman I would never forget; he pulled me out of the river and took me to the hospital. When I got there I was so psychotic they couldn't stitch up my cuts, so I returned to hospital the next day to be stitched up when I calmed down. The doctors said that I was psychotic. It took me about one and a half years to get me into hospital after that event. If I had been admitted straight away things might have been different. During this time, the first time after my drink was spiked, it took me a fortnight to get back to sleep; it was just crazy. I came across the guys who had given me the spiked pint and asked them about the incident; they admitted to spiking me.

I thought that the people who spiked me wanted me to get involved in a snuff film, but this might have been my psychosis, but I've always been wary about this when out in the town and now I always finish my drink before going to the toilet, I would never leave it lying at the bar.

I had a lot of responsibility as a 16-year-old, working in a bar. In the past I experienced very aggressive physical and sexual abuse. It started one day when I was raped by a friend of the family who worked in the same bar. Earlier in life my mum also abused me physically, scalding me, hitting with ash trays and belts; I also used to be smacked in the bath whilst naked. I think that my mum was unhappy with her life because she was single at the time with four kids. I've never discussed this with my mother. My psychologist said I should confront her, but now I think she's too old. The abuse went on for years and years, and most of the time it was only me that she attacked (my siblings did not receive the same violence from our mother). My mum was a bit of a drinker, but she was a responsible person working at the time. My real father abused my mum physically and used to beat her up. My stepdad was a different character altogether, and I was his favourite. The physical abuse was tolerable, but then I got bullied at school and began to soil myself – the bullying then got worse as a result, and I was laughed at. The sexual abuse happened from between 15 and 17 years old. Afterwards I left Newcastle to get out of the situation – I had to get out. I never told anybody about it until I was 43 or 44 years old, and when I did, the police got involved and questioned me. I found out from the police that a lot more was done by the abuser and that he was a dangerous man. The guy destroyed me; I still suffer sexual problems to this day, flashbacks, and it caused violent damage to me. I remember that he used to say sorry and gave me money afterwards. It's just that I can't get it out of my head. I know it wasn't my fault, and others who have experienced what I have and have been raped shouldn't feel dirty and should have a clean conscious. He's destroyed my sex life, but he hasn't destroyed me because I'm coming back!

During the year after the spiking experience I still managed to keep my job whilst I was still psychotic. However, I was starting to see things. As I was driving to work every morning I would see the Ku Klux Klan on the side of the road asking me whether I wanted to join them, and I would see dead bodies laying on the road. I was also smelling bad smells and tasting sulphur. All these senses – it was just me hallucinating. The tastes were bitter; the only way I can describe it was like when you drink tequila and you suck the lemon. I was hearing rustling in the back of my vehicle; it might have been a shock absorber or it could have been something in the boot such as a body. I thought the government had planted it there. I believed that the government wanted to get me for murder, so I used to stop in the middle of the carriageway or a motorway to open my boot, but there was nothing there. I had a feeling that the government was spying on me, but these days after having received CBT from my therapist, I'm 90 per cent sure it's not true, although there's still 10 per cent of me that thinks the government is keeping an eye on me. CBT helped me to question this unusual belief. I now think, 'Put surveillance on *you*? You're not special, you're like the scarlet pimpernel, and you're everywhere! To put surveillance on you would have cost £1000's!' ... that's what CBT has taught me.

The hospital where I stayed for a period was a friendly place; the nurses were different from now, because the nurses used to sit with you and have a cigarette, and it was better then than it is now. Back then, there were more students, more staff nurses – they would sit and listen to you and talk to you; there seemed to be less clinical paperwork. Nowadays, all I see is nurses with paperwork.

When I was experiencing voices, I was always up to mischief. It was terrible as the voices were always very degrading and nasty. The voices used to say to me, 'Right, see that knife on the table, put it in your sock and make sure you hurt that guy in the jugular; then you can go back to sleep and I will stop'. Later on I told the nurses about this, and I was immediately given olanzapine, which knocked me out. I was then transferred to another hospital where I was locked up to calm down; I was like a zombie for three days.

In the wards I would see nude women on the wall and a nude woman would sit beside me. I think it was linked to my sexual abuse, although it was a man who raped me and I was seeing a woman. I had a big beard, long hair, smelly clothes and the joints of my legs were sore due to poor hygiene, but the staff weren't really bothered. I was only eight stone. I was on a crash diet, drinking Diet Coke because I was trying to fit through a window to get out of the hospital. I was depressed for two years; electroconvulsive therapy was the last resort. Before the CBT was offered to me I was only taking medication and the pills made me feel shit and made me sleep constantly; I didn't get any benefit from them.

When I had CBT I remember that my therapist wrote on a blackboard and helped me to think about the evidence for and against some of my beliefs. On the blackboard we wrote about the plus side and the minus side of the evidence.

I recall one time when I wasn't in hospital I was going to kill my girlfriend because the voices were telling me to kill her. I would have been sectioned if I had told anybody. I decided that I was going to make a Bolognese sauce with 300 to 400 paracetamol pills and mix it up, but I ditched that idea and put it in the bin.

The CBT taught me where the voices came from – they came from the abuse and the drink spiking and the psychosis; it wasn't my fault – it was just one of these things. Luckily I've had a therapist to help me and get me out of hospital when I was starting to feel well again.

I also recall another day when I was chasing aliens with a knife and hitting trees. I thought the aliens were trees. I hadn't taken my medication for about five days and I was drinking all the time. I hope there will be a day in my life when I will be medication free. I will try to continue to do my CBT homework, and as long as I do my homework, I hope that I will eventually be medication free. It is important to me that I will be medication free one day.

My CBT homework was to listen to the audio recordings of my CBT sessions as often as possible, as they told you what to do, how to do it, what not to do. The one bit of CBT which stuck with me when I was told not to blame myself because the person who abused me was a man in power: 'he was a friend of the family so I couldn't talk to my family because they wouldn't have believed me'. My homework was to keep working on the pros on cons of my beliefs about people on phones talking about me, people driving in the street surveilling me and people in hospital trying to kill me. I kept on working at it.

I looked at the pros and cons of the voices with my therapist. He told me for the first time where the voices came from. I'd never asked that question before; I was frightened to ask it because I thought they (the government) had planted something (a microchip) in my brain that was giving me the voices to self-harm. I used to sit in the hospital room and smash cups; and then I would cut myself. This experience was like taking lorazepam. I would just sit there chilling, thinking, 'Yeah, brilliant no voices' whilst I cut my wrists. Self-harm was the only way I coped when the voices were strong until I had CBT. Once I started CBT I would listen back to the audio recordings of my previous CBT sessions and answer the voices back, which is a great thing. You don't say to them, 'You're a bastard, I'm going to punch your head' as the voices only get worse. You've got to be calm and collective about it; when talking back to your voices you've got to say, 'Fair enough'. When I did this the voices would say to me, 'You're a useless person', but in response I would say, 'I've got friends, my 50th birthday will be full of good women and good men and I'm a good guy. I'm not useless. I used to be a tailor. I've done mental health support work for people with autism so I'm not a useless guy and I make people happy'. After that the voices usually stayed quiet for weeks at a time. I'm thankful that I've got audio recordings of my CBT sessions, they are like gold dust!

My tip for successfully engaging in CBT is that you really need to do the homework; be in a zone with a cup of tea or juice – no caffeine, no alcohol – and just listen to your therapy audio recordings. The voices used to say, 'You're a useless person, you're scum', and I say, 'No I'm not, people love me'. The voices flared up in reaction to this. I would respond by saying, 'I don't care what you are saying. I will talk to you when I'm ready'. This was a mental breakthrough. I'd like to get out there and tell everybody. I think CBT would work for everybody who does their homework and listens to their audio recordings and talks calmly back to the voices.

I said to my dad before he died from cancer that all I want to do is work, settle down and get a job, and I've done this.

Summary of Key Coping Techniques: Dos and Don't from David

For everyone who has mental illness, I would say give CBT a go; don't let anybody distract you.

Do ... your homework. It reminds you of the conversations you have had with your therapist and you can work on it. I know that I can listen to my therapy audio recordings and I will be in top form when I return for my next therapy session.

Dealing with Visions

Robert Dudley, Rea Cheetham, Samuel Sargeant, and
Daniel Collerton

Key Points

1. Visions are common.
2. How you make sense of your vision is important as to whether the vision is upsetting.
3. Unhelpful coping can make visions worse.
4. Helpful coping can reduce the upset visions cause.
5. It is important to talk to others about your visions.
6. You can change the way you make sense of the visions and what you do to cope.
7. Using these methods, visions can become less frequent or people can find effective ways to manage them.

Introduction

Some people frequently see things that other people cannot, an experience called a visual hallucination, or vision. Visions are not as common as auditory hallucinations (or hearing voices) seem to be in psychosis. Perhaps two-thirds of people with psychosis hear voices, whereas it is more like a quarter or a third will have seen a vision. We asked people with visions what it was that they saw. They told us that their visions mainly involved seeing a face or a person, and less often it was an animal or an object. We also asked people how they felt when they saw the vision. Some, but not all, found the vision to be a distressing experience. We think the amount of distress experienced is partly a result of how people make sense of or understand their visions. For example, if they think the vision can cause harm to them or to someone they care about, it can be a very frightening experience. As a result of this, they may look for ways to take care of themselves; for example, they may hide away from the vision.

There has been relatively little research into why people see things that others do not, so we don't really know why it happens. Almost certainly there will be different causes and factors for different people. We know, for example, that people with migraines and epilepsy report seeing things. Whether this occurs for the same reasons as in psychosis is unclear, but the more extensive research on voices in people with psychosis may help provide some ideas. It is thought that in some cases, people hear voices as they mistake their own inner speech for an external voice. Inner speech is what you hear in your head when you read, or when you are thinking to yourself. At first it seems unlikely that you could confuse this internal experience for another person's voice, as it would seem obvious that you can tell when you have heard something externally or when you have thought something to yourself.

However, if you think for a moment about inner speech it can at times be quite different from your usual inner voice. Just for a moment listen to your inner voice saying something like your name and address, now try imagining a distinctive voice like Darth Vader's, or a familiar voice like that of your mum or dad saying the same thing. This shows that you can hear things in your mind that sound quite different from your usual inner voice. If we had such an experience and did not recognise that this was our own inner voice, it is entirely possible that we may think it was coming from outside our heads, because we know it has to come from somewhere!

How does this help us understand why some people see things? Well, the basic idea is the same as with voices, that for some reason we are not recognising our own internal experiences and instead we think that the experience is coming from the world around us. The difference is that it is not our own inner speech that we confuse with a real voice; rather it seems that people with visions may be mistaking their own mental imagery for real perceptions. Mental imagery is seeing with the mind's eye, or the ability to picture things in our own mind.

It is strange to think of us hearing or seeing things as a result of us mistaking where the sound or image came from. Our senses are so powerful that if we see or hear something, then we believe it must be true. 'Seeing is believing', as they say.

However, this explanation of hallucinations actually fits quite well with how we think people perceive the world around them. One way to understand it is that our brains do not work like a video camera by capturing the world around us and sending these images to our brains. We have found out from trying to get robots and computers to 'see' the world using video cameras that this is a difficult task if we only rely on pictures and images from a camera. So we have had to teach computers to work like our brains do and use helpful shortcuts to speed things up. Essentially, the brain builds a picture in the mind of what we expect to see, and this expectation is checked against what our eyes and senses tell us. So we develop a picture of the world around us by combining different sources of information from the world, as well as checking this against what we expect to see. If you look at Figure 11.1 it will help to explain what we mean.

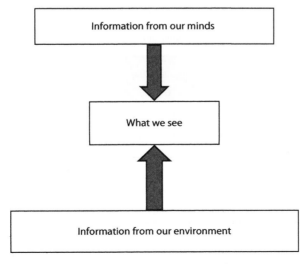

Figure 11.1 An illustration of the way we expect to see things and what we actually perceive, helps us to form a picture of what we then see

So how we see the world is based on a combination of what we expect to see and information from the world around us. Although this works pretty well most of the time, it can go wrong occasionally. If you think of the millions of scenes, words, objects and people we see, it is actually quite surprising it does not happen more often. Sometimes, though our mind plays tricks on us and we fall for optical illusions, and sometimes we have fleeting hallucinations. This is normal.

We think that four things can affect our chance of seeing things: (1) we can have problems with the information coming in; (2) we can have problems with our expectations of the world; (3) we can have difficulties deciding what is real or imagined; and (4) we can have strains on our judgement systems, meaning we make the wrong decision. We will explore each of these explanations in a bit more detail below, but the key message is that we can understand what leads people to have visions. Understanding this can help us 'turn down' our visions. For example, a simple thing like improving the lighting can be helpful in 'turning down' the frequency or number of visions.

Information Coming in from the Environment

Taking each of these in turn, obviously, if the information coming in from the environment is not good, our ability to check the pictures in our mind can be affected. When this happens, our brain has to work harder to make sure it does not miss important information and so it compensates for this lack of information from the world around us. If there is very little information coming in, for example, if people sit for a long time in the dark, then they will often hallucinate. There is also a condition called Charles Bonnet syndrome (CBS) that happens when people have eye disease and start losing their sight. People with CBS often report seeing visions. We have tried to illustrate this in Figure 11.2. You will notice that the arrow from the information in the environment is thin, meaning it does not provide as much information as we need, so the brain works harder and uses expectation more (which is shown by the thicker arrow). So when it is dark or we have poor vision, this can increase our chance of hallucinations.

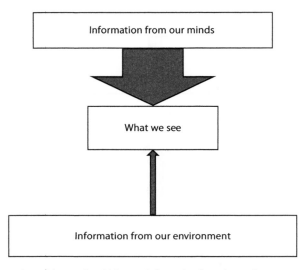

Figure 11.2 An illustration of the way in which poor information from the environment can lead to a greater need for our brain to use expectation

Sometimes this expectation can be greater, not because of problems with the information coming in, but because of recent events. If we have recently lost a family member following a bereavement, then our brain may take time to process this loss and so it expects to still see the person. For the first month or two after we have lost someone we naturally expect to see them, as this is what we have been used to for years. When we walk into a room we may assume we will see the person sitting in their chair watching the TV. This powerful expectation means that it is normal to have a strong sense that the person is in the room, and we may hear the person call our name or we may even see them for a while after they have passed away.

Some people seem to have very vivid internal imagery, which can mean that their imagination can seem very real and lifelike. This can increase the risk of confusion between what is actually happening in the real world and what we think we are seeing. When we talk to people with visions, they often report that they are creative and that their imagination is very vivid. For instance, they will often report being able to imagine characters from films or TV very clearly and to imagine what happened to these characters once the film was over. They also report very vivid dreams and that sometimes when they wake up they are not sure if the dream was real or if they are still dreaming. So although this is just anecdotal evidence, it does seem to fit with the idea that people with visions have greater creativity and more of a vivid imagination and that sometimes they may find the border between real and imagined experiences harder to tell apart. So in some ways the factors that lead to the experience of having visions could be a good thing (the ability to have rich and vivid mental imagery), but, of course, you can have too much of a good thing.

Our Expectations of the World

The power of expectation may also help explain why we tend to see faces and people when we have hallucinations, which is what people most often say they see. From a young age we develop incredible abilities in recognising faces because it really helps if we can recognise people quickly and accurately, but this leaves us at risk of seeing faces where they don't actually exist. For example, we may see faces in patterns on a carpet or wallpaper, or we may see faces when we look at clouds in the sky. It shows how we are really good at seeing faces where they don't actually exist. So if you were going to make any mistakes about your visual perception, there is a good chance it would be that you would see a face or a person.

As we have said, our visual system is actually pretty good at deciding whether something is real or imagined. We generally don't confuse real events for imagined ones. Sometimes, though, because we are tired or stressed, our ability to make this decision may change, and this can lead to us making more mistakes. Chris Ryan, the Special Air Service (SAS) solider, provides a good example of this happening. He was under huge strain, fleeing from the Iraqi army in the Gulf War, and had not slept properly for days. He reported seeing his wife and daughter out in the desert. So at certain points when we are stressed or tired we may confuse imaginary and real experiences.

Difficulty Deciding on What is Real or Imagined

Sometimes our visual system can make mistakes not because of huge stress like being in a war, but just because it can vary at certain times in our day. Each day as we fall asleep or wake up, the boundary between reality and imagination blurs. Two of the authors of this chapter have had the experience of seeing things at that point between waking and sleeping that they later realised were not real. This is very common. We know as well that if people are deprived of sleep for a few days or more they often report visions.

Given the way our perceptual system works, it is not that unusual to have odd experiences like seeing things. As we said before, not everyone who sees things finds them upsetting, and we know that some people like having such experiences and will take hallucinogenic drugs for this purpose.

However, when people see things that are not real and they do not have an explanation, they can get pretty upset. Even people with Charles Bonnet Syndrome who know they are losing their sight can still get very worried when they have visions. Sometimes people see really frightening things, or things that remind them of frightening times, or they think the vision is going to have a bad consequence; like they will lose their mind, or get locked up, or they fear that the vision will interfere with their life so much that they cannot do anything else. They worry they will not be able to cope.

But none of these things have to be true. Lots of people live well with their hallucinations. CBT can help you understand why you are having these experiences, why they are frightening you and it can help you find ways of making sure that you understand the reality behind those fears.

It seems that for people with visions there are three main reasons they become upset about seeing things. For some people seeing a vision feels like a threat to their physical or psychological safety. If they see a vision, they may fear that they are going to be hurt or it is a sign that they are going mad. For other people it is the actual content of what they see that really upsets them, even if they know it is a hallucination. For others it is the fact that the visions have not gone away and they keep interfering with daily life that really distresses them. Usually people try hard to manage these experiences, but the way they try and cope can sometimes make the situation worse.

We have to be honest and say we are really limited in knowing what is the best way to help people cope with visions. Most of what we know has been learnt from talking to people with visions and asking them what they do to cope with these experiences, as well as case studies that have used cognitive therapy for people with visions. So what we do know is that strategies that can help, include changing or improving the quality of the information coming into the senses. So it may help, for instance, to use brighter lighting. Another helpful strategy is to break the line of sight so people may blink or look away for a while and reset their perceptual system.

People can also look out for common patterns or triggers for their visions. Falling asleep or waking up are times when the boundary between real and imagined can become blurred. Being sleepy or stressed or changes to the internal system caused by taking alcohol or drugs can be recognised as factors that lead to the experience of seeing visions. Also, heightened expectation, such as being on the lookout for the experience at a certain time of day, can increase the chance of seeing it. For example, you may have had the experience of waiting for a visitor or a delivery and then repeatedly think you have heard the doorbell only to find no one is there. That is the power of expectation.

Putting all these things together, it would seem that visions may be more common when:
we are tired,
when we are stressed,
when we have not slept well,

when we are expecting to see the vision,

when it is dark,

when we have been drinking.

All of these things challenge the perceptual system and our ability to judge what is internal or external in origin. Changing some of these may help reduce how often you see things.

Of course, you can know things with your head but not feel them to be true. If a person still thinks that seeing a vision means they may be hurt, we have to help them realise that seeing is not the same as believing and that the vision is harmless, a trick of the mind, and it cannot hurt them. To help find out if it is real we may get the person to throw a scrunched-up piece of paper at the vision, or try and take a photo of it and then think about whether this shows it is real or not. If someone finds the content of the vision really upsetting, we can help people distract themselves from the content, or even try and change it so that it is no longer so upsetting. We can do this by getting people to stay with the image rather than trying to get rid of it quickly. It is tempting not to think about or pay attention to the image but this can sometimes make things worse so we need to help the person find out that the image can become less fearful if we 'stay' with it. A bit like watching a horror film many times over, by the 100th time it might actually be quite boring.

Regardless of the exact nature of the experience, there are some key and important messages that need to be reinforced:

It is not real.

At times everyone's eyes play tricks on them.

It cannot harm you.

You have not lost your mind.

You are safe.

You are normal.

We will illustrate next how we have used this understanding to help two people with visions.

Strains on Our Judgement Systems

A Simple Example

Joanna is a 25-year-old woman who is studying hard for her final exams at College; she is working long hours and is feeling increasingly stressed. Whilst revising late at night in her flat she started to see her grandfather sitting in an armchair in her room. Joanna's grandfather had passed away two years earlier. Joanna had a close relationship with him. Seeing her grandfather seemed incredibly real and was very confusing for Joanna. She was not afraid of the vision, as it was her grandfather who she loved, but she began to fear that she was losing her mind and became very worried that she would start talking to him.

Why Has This New Visual Hallucination Emerged?

During periods of stress in her life Joanna's grandfather had been very supportive. This was the first period of stress that Joanna had to face without her grandfather. Perhaps then it is not surprising that she would see him during this time. During periods of bereavement people often report seeing their loved one. It is likely that our expectation to see them in familiar places will influence our perceptual system.

Table 11.1 An example of how Joanna understood her vision

Situation	Thoughts	Response
Late at night revising and see my grandfather in the armchair.	There is something wrong with me. I'm losing my mind.	Don't tell anyone, Worry

It may be helpful for Joanna to develop an understanding of this experience that is less distressing for her. Researchers have shown that people become upset with visual hallucinations owing to the way(s) in which they make sense of them (Gauntlett-Gilbert & Kuipers, 2005). Within cognitive therapy we work hard to develop an alternative explanation to reduce the upset caused by the visual hallucination. We do this with the person by looking at the situation, the thoughts that run through their mind and how they respond. An example of a distressing interpretation of the vision is provided in Table 11.1.

To help consider an alternative, less distressing explanation, it may be useful for Joanna to learn that under similar conditions other people have had similar experiences. So we may share information like 'More than one million adults in Britain, while awake, repeatedly see people, animals, or objects that appear real but are not visible to others' (Collerton et al. 2005, p. 737). Just acknowledging the strain that Joanna's perceptual system (stress, late nights, lack of sleep) has been placed under may help her to recognise that under certain conditions her eyes can make mistakes.

We would help Joanna understand that our visual perceptual system works from a combination of information coming into it from the world around us and our expectation of seeing certain things in specific situations. We have seen that the chance of making mistakes is increased when the information coming in is of poor quality. Joanna was studying in a dimly lit room, and her grandfather always appeared in the shadows of her standing lamp. Also she was under high levels of stress and getting little sleep, which also leads to our perceptual system becoming strained (a bit like in Figure 11.2).

Knowing about why we see things may help Joanna change the triggers to this experience. She could:

- Change the layout of her room; move the armchair and the standing lamp.
- Improve the lighting in the room.

It is also important for her to recognise that she may be under stress and that seeing her grandfather is a way of her mind telling her that she needs to take care of herself. To this end she may be encouraged to:

- Introduce a good sleep routine; taking steps to prepare the mind and body for sleep, have a relaxing bath on an evening, reduce caffeine intake and ensure that her bedroom is a comfortable temperature.
- Develop a good study timetable; stop studying until the early hours of the morning.
- Introduce some ways to cope with stress, such as increasing her exercise, spending time with her friends and reintroducing an old hobby or interest.

What Can a Carer/Friend Do?

If you are a carer of someone like Joanna, it can feel puzzling that your loved one is having these unusual experiences. However, it is important that these experiences are talked about in order to help understand them and manage them better. Don't be afraid to talk about them with the person. Help the person look for patterns and triggers to the experience. Encourage them to look after themselves, get some sleep and not to overwork. Perhaps you can see that they are pushing themselves too hard in a way that they cannot, so your help in gently supporting them to slow down and take care of themselves will be important.

> **A More Complex Example**
>
> Max is an 18-year-old man who has recently started to see what he calls a spirit. This started when Max moved in with his girlfriend. Max was terrified of the spirit and hid in the bathroom whenever he saw it. Max believed that the spirit could physically harm him.

Why Has This New Visual Hallucination Emerged?

Max and his girlfriend moved into a flat on an estate, and one evening Max was assaulted by some youths whilst walking to the local pub. Max had been badly bullied at school and as a young adult was mugged and attacked whilst walking home late at night. This first assault had left him critically ill, and he had needed lengthy rehabilitation to recover from his injuries. The recent assault was very traumatic for Max, and he began to feel unsafe even in his new home. His sleep became disturbed, and he was fearful of leaving the flat. As with Joanna, in CBT we would ask what Max makes of his experience using the format below.

Max needs support to help him learn that his vision isn't a threat to his safety but may be a sign that he is feeling unsafe owing to the assaults he has experienced. At first it may be unhelpful to directly question the reality of this experience, as for Max the vision is very real. One task may be to help him notice that he sees the vision late at night, when it is dark and he is tired. He sees it when he feels more vulnerable and at risk. It is important for him to be able to see this link. To help with this we may ask him to record when he sees the vision (using Table 11.2) to help establish the link between how he is feeling and the presence of the vision. This may help Max realise that the vision is a way of telling him that he is feeling vulnerable and scared. Rather than be upset at this, he can learn to acknowledge this feeling and understand it is a normal reaction that many people feel after being a victim of an assault.

It may help Max if he could establish a different night-time routine and perhaps not stay up so late. He would be encouraged to share his experience with his girlfriend, who could support him when this experience happens; this will help Max feel that he doesn't have to face these experiences alone. In order to help Max overcome his fear of the vision, he needs to learn that he is safe. Max's girlfriend may help Max by encouraging him to try the following:

- Can Max observe his girlfriend's reactions when the spirit is present? If he is not sure about telling her about these experiences, he could start by observing how their pet cat reacts to the spirit. This may help him establish if others can see it or not.
- If he begins to doubt if it is real, maybe he could he try staying in the room with the spirit with the support of his girlfriend?

Table 11.2 An example of how Max understood his vision

Situation	Thoughts	Response
Staying up watching TV late at night, on my own, and see the spirit.	It is real, it is here to hurt me and the spirit will attack me.	Feel scared, hide in the bathroom and lock the door.

- If Max was willing and felt safe enough he could try shining a torch onto the spirit to establish what happens? Is the image translucent? Is there a shadow? What would this mean about it being a real figure?
- Could Max try taking a photograph of the spirit? What's in the photo? All of these may help Max establish that the vision is not real. If it is not real, it cannot hurt him.

It is likely that Max and his girlfriend would benefit from professional support, such as a CBT therapist and care team to guide this work.

Summary of Key CBT Techniques: The Dos and Don'ts

Dos	Don'ts
• Talk with someone about your experiences. • Recognise that the brain can easily make mistakes. Hallucinations or visual distortions are common experiences. • Question the explanation you make of these experiences. Check out what a friend or family member thinks of this idea. • Watch other people's responses when the vision is there or try to take a picture of it.	• Isolate yourself or deal with these experiences alone. • Rely on substances to cope with this experience. • Don't stay up late. Try and establish a good sleep pattern. • Don't be afraid to talk to your family, or friends so you are not facing this alone. • Don't be afraid to talk to you GP to find out if more help may be available to you.

References

Collerton, D., Perry, E. & McKeith, I. (2005) Why people see things that are not there: A novel perception and attention deficit model for recurrent complex visual hallucinations. *Behavioral and Brain Sciences*, 28, 737–94.

Gauntlett-Gilbert, J. & Kuipers, E. (2005) Visual hallucinations in psychiatric conditions: Appraisals and their relationship to distress. *British Journal of Clinical Psychology*, 44, 77–87.

Further Reading

For more information about visions please consider the following.

Websites/Other Info

A website which provides examples of when people have seen faces in everyday objects: www.boredpanda.com/pareidolia-faces-everyday-objects/

Useful website information includes Michael Shermer's TED talk covering topics that show how powerful expectation can be and how easily tricked we can be by optical illusions, etc.: www.ted.com/talks/michael_shermer_on_believing_strange_things?language=en

Intervoice is an online community where people share experiences about hearing voices, but they often consider other experiences such as visions: www.intervoiceonline.org

12 Compassion-Focused Approaches for Clients, Families and Health Care Providers

Charles Heriot-Maitland, Eleanor Longden, Katherine Elliott, Suzanne Bell, Paul Gilbert and Nicola P. Wright

Key Points

1. Use your understanding of our three emotion systems (threat, soothing and drive) to apply compassion-focused approaches for your loved one to decrease distressing emotions and increase soothing, connection and progress toward goals.
2. Use compassion-focused principles and approaches to reduce distressing emotions in the family and/or health care environment.
3. Use compassion-focused exercises to calm yourself and connect with others in order to provide 'care for the carer'.

Introduction

Psychosis is linked with difficulties in coping with distressing emotions and processing threat. Given the important role of emotion in psychosis, techniques derived from compassion-focused therapy (CFT) can offer beneficial ways for coping with threat/fear as well as distressing emotions more generally. The theoretical underpinning of CFT focuses on three emotion regulation systems: (1) the drive system (e.g., feelings of being motivated or excited and achieving goals); (2) the threat system (e.g., feelings of anger, anxiety or disgust); and (3) the soothing system (e.g., feelings of safety, contentment, connectedness and soothing). Research on CFT has shown it to be a viable and acceptable treatment for those with psychosis and is linked to reducing the symptoms of depression and enhancing self-esteem (Braehler et al. 2013).

Individuals with psychosis may often experience voices and/or distressing beliefs as critical and threatening. These experiences, when combined with stigma (both from others, but also beliefs the person has about themselves), can create a vicious cycle of shame, self-criticism, low mood and social isolation. When the threat system is active in this way, it can be difficult to feel motivated and/or to feel safe and connected with others. As such, CFT can help individuals activate the soothing/affiliative emotional system in order to cope better with perceived threats (i.e., to regulate the threat system) whilst continuing to increase motivation (i.e., the drive system). One way in which CFT can help with activating the soothing system is by enhancing connecting relationships with others. In this way, we can still experience threat but not let it prevent us from pursuing valued goals or from building important relationships with others. Compassion-focused approaches can help reduce the severity and impact of the symptoms of psychosis and likewise help individuals change the relationship they have with their voices or distressing experiences and thoughts. In addition, CFT can help find greater meaning in, and understanding of, one's experiences and thus provide the right psychological conditions to engage in meaningful activities and goals. Ultimately, the principles and practice of compassion-focused approaches can help distressed individuals reduce feelings of fear and threat and, through increased self-soothing and connection, enhance the ability to live a more meaningful life. This chapter outlines how CFT can help (1) individuals who experience psychosis, (2) their family members and carers, (3) their treatment team and (4) the larger society.

Personal Disclosure (NW)

When I was in my early 20s I was looking for part-time employment to help fund my university degree. I applied to several jobs but received very few interviews and no job offers from the interviews that I attended. This process went on for several months. As the weeks progressed I became more and more down on myself and fearful that I would never find a job and end up with significant debt. This self-criticism and fear seeped into other domains of my life as well. At university, something that I always did well in, I began to question my abilities and worry about performing well on exams. I also worried that my friends and family thought less of me because I was unable to secure employment.

I noticed myself going down this rabbit hole of self-deprecating, semi-paranoid thoughts when a planned family function came up and I started taking steps to avoid going to it. In calling to mind an image of this event, I realised that my sense of shame from being unemployed was fuelling my critical inner voice and that the negative thoughts I was having about myself, and that I perceived others to have about me, were not based in reality. I specifically pictured my grandmother welcoming me with open arms and smothering me with comfort and praise. Seeing myself through my grandmother's eyes provided me with an overwhelming feeling of warmth and compassion. This image enabled me to approach the job search process more openly and mindfully, with a more balanced self-representation.

This personal experience helps to highlight several broader issues in relation to self-compassion:

1. Our minds are sensitive to perceiving threats. In turn, early difficult or traumatic life experiences can increase this sensitivity.
2. When triggered by external factors, worries and fears can compound one another and spiral out of control.
3. Distressing emotions such as shame and self-criticism can lead to avoidance, reduce connections with other people and increase distressing thoughts and emotions.
4. Using compassion-focused approaches can help reduce distressing emotions such as fear and self-critical thoughts, leading to a reduction of perceived threat, lower bodily arousal and a greater sense of calmness and safety.
5. Thinking and acting with compassion can help calm us, create healing internal environments and free us up from distressing thoughts and emotions in order to work toward and achieve meaningful goals.

Positive Aspects of Distressing Voices, Visions and Beliefs

A large percentage of individuals with lived experience of psychosis have encountered adverse and traumatic life events, such as childhood abuse and bullying. Correspondingly, it is increasingly recognised that so-called psychotic symptoms such as voices, visions or unusual beliefs may be linked to difficult or unprocessed emotions. As such, applying compassion-based approaches to reduce feelings of threat, fear and distress can create the necessary feelings of safety to begin the process of 'unpacking' the real-life problems and adversities associated with distressing experiences. For example, if a voice is telling a person that it is not safe to leave the house, then the message could be seen as a cue to check in regarding how safe one feels and what steps we can take to care for ourselves in order to feel safer and continue with our day-to-day life. Through compassion, soothing and finding meaning in one's experiences, it can often be possible to change the relationship with the experience itself, whether a voice, vision or distressing belief, so that it becomes less threatening. CFT can help calm the threat system so one can work through past difficulties, find healing and ultimately live a fuller and more meaningful life. With practice, many voice hearers find their voices can become less critical and more companionable. In turn, distressing beliefs may diminish as the individual engages in activities that are more consistent with their values and goals.

Taking a Compassionate Approach

Three-Circles Model of Emotion

As discussed previously, CFT focuses on three emotion regulation systems: (1) the drive system (e.g., feelings of being driven or excited and resource seeking); (2) the threat system (e.g., feelings of anger, anxiety or disgust); and (3) the self-soothing or contentment system (e.g., feelings of safety, connectedness and soothing).

Social Context and Relationships

CFT aims to create the conditions within a person's body, mind and social environment that will provide the best chance of integrating and working with distressing emotions and experiences. In this section, we will be focusing on the social environment, with an emphasis on exploring the role of relationships, interactions and social contexts in creating these 'optimum' conditions for recovery.

A good place to start in understanding the role of relationships in emotional wellbeing is by observing the behaviour of infants when they are born. John Bowlby, the 'founding father' of attachment theory, studied numerous infant-parent interactions and concluded that all human infants are born with a natural instinct to seek closeness with a caregiver and to feel safeness when that figure is close – effectively that our brains are 'wired up' to feel comforted in the face of loving, caring and kindness. It is natural for humans – in fact, very much part of our evolutionary make-up – to feel soothed by caring, attachment and nurturing from others. In CFT language, what this means is that experiences of closeness, connection and social safeness have a natural (built-in) calming effect on the threat system, as well as activating the soothing system. See Figure 12.1 below.

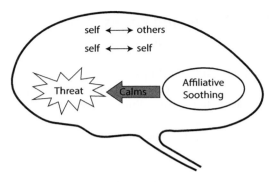

Figure 12.1 The benefits of soothing on the stress system.

Therefore when a person's experiences are often characterised by high threat system activation – as is the case in psychosis – there is potentially a key role for social connections and relationships in calming this system down. Another important insight from Bowlby's model of attachment is that this experience of closeness and safeness with a parent/caregiver also acts as a secure base for a child when growing up, effectively providing a kind of platform from which the child can develop the confidence and courage to begin venturing out into the world, exploring, taking risks, etc. Again, we can draw a parallel here with the experience of psychosis, in that there is potentially an important role for social connections in helping people develop the confidence and courage to start exploring their own experiences (e.g., distressing voices, visions, beliefs).

Social relationships may therefore have a dual role in psychosis recovery – as a threat calmer and a secure base, both of which can help a person develop a more constructive relationship with difficult experiences and emotions. This gives rise to two main questions: (1) What can you, as an individual, do to improve your experiences of social safeness? and (2) What can the people around you do to help improve it? To answer these questions, we will look at three different levels of relationships and social contexts that may be important to people with psychosis: friends and family, mental health staff and services, and communities and societies.

Friends and Family

It can understandably be very distressing to witness a friend or loved one experiencing unusual perceptions and beliefs. This can often leave those closest to that person feeling worried and confused themselves, and in their fear and uncertainty (of, for example, not knowing what to do for the best), family and friends might inadvertently create an atmosphere of tension and heightened emotion. Again, this is understandable and, in CFT terms, is exactly what we'd expect to happen when our evolved threat system becomes activated. It's not anyone's fault. However, it is clear that this is not an ideal social experience for helping a distressed person access their soothing system or for helping to create a 'secure base' to begin exploring and understanding what is happening to them. So although these common reactions from family and friends are understandable in the situation, the kinds of social interactions that would probably be most helpful in these difficult times are likely to be those involving calmness, listening, understanding and validation.

Mental Health Staff and Services

As with experiences of family and friends, those accessing mental health services are likely to find some interactions that feel unhelpful (e.g., staff who seem stressed, detached, cold, etc.). For those working within mental health services, the three circles model can provide a useful framework for raising awareness about how they feel they are functioning in their work (and home) life. For instance, the mental health professional could ask themselves the following: How are my three systems balanced as I go about my job? Which system is usually most dominant? Which could do with more building up? What balance of the three systems would be most helpful for me (my own emotional health), as well as for me to create the kinds of interactions and experiences that are most helpful for the people using our services?

The three circles model is not only a helpful roadmap towards improving emotional balance at the personal level (i.e., self and clients), but also in understanding how these emotional contexts are being activated at a mental health service level. For instance, it may be useful to think about the three circles in your own mental health team. Is your service operating from the threat system? What is the influence of the drive system? How can we help move it more towards the soothing system? Services operating in their threat systems might, for example, have dominant cultures of things like risk assessment, enforced drug treatment, and use of more authoritarian procedures and powers. For example, acute inpatient units can be very threat- and protection-focused environments, with locked doors, alarms sounding and high levels of distress for both patients and staff. In terms of the three circles model, there is serious potential for an imbalance within such an environment, with a risk of sustained high threat and reduced opportunities to foster positive and soothing experiences.

Often the dominance of the threat system extends beyond the individual mental health unit/team and into the structure and hierarchy of the organisation. Again, this is not anyone's fault; conversely, a focus on creating calmer, nurturing and safer environments for staff and service users has the potential to provide a much stronger foundation for working therapeutically with distressing emotions and experiences.

Communities and Societies

The scope of the CFT model extends beyond individuals, families and services into communities and society as a whole. For instance, we know that a lot of the threat experience associated with psychosis comes from the social stigma around psychiatric diagnoses like 'schizophrenia'. This stigma brings an additional layer of threat linked to one's social position (i.e., the threat of social rejection and devaluation). Many of those diagnosed with schizophrenia/psychosis internalise these stigmatising views from society, which can lead to self-stigma and shame (internal threat). One of the great challenges is how to create more understanding communities where difficult experiences can be expressed, explored and safely discussed without fear of negative social judgement and other adverse consequences. The media has a considerable responsibility given that psychosis is frequently portrayed as dangerous and frightening. These messages, of course, negatively shape attitudes and can reduce the public's confidence in being able to engage calmly and compassionately with those who experience mental health difficulties.

An antidote to this are numerous community-based organisations that offer safe and validating peer support. One example is the Hearing Voices Movement (HVM), which operates via national Hearing Voices Networks and is coordinated internationally via the charity Intervoice (www.intervoiceonline.org). Via peer-led groups and meetings, the HVM's initiatives can offer the kind of connecting experiences that activate the soothing system and facilitate exploring and dealing with feelings of fear and threat. However, much more can be done to enhance feelings of safety and reduce threat, such as educating the general public, sharing personal stories and raising awareness. In CFT, we have tried to provide more positive representation by sharing the story of a young man's journey to developing a compassionate relationship with his voices. This video, is a five-minute animation called 'Compassion for Voices' (http://compassionforvoices.com/videos/compassion-for-voices-film/), which is freely available on YouTube. Can more of us find the courage to share our personal stories? It requires courage and support, yet providing the opportunities to do so has the potential to help our communities and societies to feel safer, more confident and better equipped to offer compassionate listening and support.

An Example of Activating Compassion towards Critical Voices

Bob is a 21-year-old young man who hears voices. They often tell him that others are 'out to get him' and that it's 'not safe' to leave his home. As a result, Bob has moved into the basement and covered up the windows to prevent others from being able to see him. Although he used to enjoy cycling and playing football with his friends, his fear of both his voices and of being harmed by others has led him to give up these activities. The more he stays in his basement, the worse his mood becomes. He feels sad and lonely and increasingly spends more and more time in bed.

Questions

1. Based on the three-circle model outlined earlier, which emotion-regulation system has been activated?
2. What could Bob, a carer/friend or mental health professional do to help Bob improve his mood?

Based on our previous discussion, Bob's threat system appears to be activated. It makes sense that if Bob is being told by his voices that it is not safe to leave his home that he would remain indoors and try to hide. As his time at home increases and his valued activities decrease, it makes sense that his mood would also deteriorate, creating a vicious cycle of low mood and increased fear, in which he is never able to check out whether or not it is safe to leave his home.

Understanding this process (i.e., as a process that makes sense) is the first step for a friend/carer or health care worker to help support Bob. By approaching Bob with compassionate understanding, this can increase a safe and therapeutic relationship for Bob to be able to express why he is remaining at home. Compassionate relationships can help to activate the soothing system and help Bob feel less threatened and increase his drive. For Bob, understanding this process himself is the first step to regaining a sense of control in his life, which very likely feels out of control. By understanding what is happening, he can begin to engage in exercises that can help to activate self-soothing, which in turn will help him begin to take valued action (e.g., begin to leave the house, eventually engaging in activities that he used to enjoy). Ultimately, this can help reduce the threat system and increase his drive. Table 12.1 provides an example of what Bob may be feeling and thinking.

Table 12.1 Linking triggers to emotions, thoughts and behaviours.

Situation/trigger	Emotions (which system is activated?)	Thoughts	Behaviours (what did I do?)
Voices telling Bob that it is dangerous to leave his home.	Fear (threat system activated).	If I leave my home, people will try to harm me.	Stay at home (drive system reduced).

This approach can be used by all people involved (carers/friends and mental health professionals as well) to help support Bob. For example, a family member may not understand why Bob is hiding in the basement and become fearful for his wellbeing (i.e., threat system activated), which may lead to thoughts of 'Something is wrong!' or 'This can't be happening!' or 'What do I do?'. This can lead to frustration and possibly even arguments with Bob to try to get him to 'snap out of it', which, although completely understandable, may not be the most helpful response. Mental health professionals may also see Bob and think 'I need to make him better', which may lead to increased anxiety at one's own ability to do this (i.e., increased threat) or, conversely, increased drive in wanting to give Bob too many activities to do because they think the activities will help him to improve. Again, these may be well intentioned, but may not be the most helpful when Bob's threat system is activated. By understanding our own emotion-regulation systems, we can better understand each other and be in a better position to be compassionate in our approach to offering help.

Take a moment to fill out your own experience, whether you are experiencing voices or distressing beliefs, or whether you are a friend/carer or mental health professional offering assistance to someone who is having distressing experiences in Table 12.2.

Table 12.2 Exercise on linking triggers to emotions, thoughts and behaviours.

Situation/trigger	Emotions (which system is activated?)	Thoughts	Behaviours (what did I do?)

Compassion-Focused Exercises to Calm Our Body, Mind and Emotions

Here we outline a number of compassion-focused approaches for compassionate attention, thinking, reasoning, feeling, sensing, imagery and behaviour. Just like exercise and a healthy diet are important for our wellbeing, the benefits of compassion-focused exercises develop over time and with ongoing practice. These approaches are like a vitamin rather than a pain killer: we may not notice the benefits at first, but over time these compassion-focused exercises can change our brain, body, thinking and experiences. Just as we would not expect that exercise would show results the first time (in fact we may feel pain exerting muscles we have not used in a long time), compassion-focused exercises are not a 'one shot deal'. They require ongoing practice, just like an exercise regimen or healthy eating. CFT is an important approach, given our evolutionary built-in tendency to look for, or 'attend' to, threat and to notice our mistakes. The human brain has a default mode that allows us to focus on a number of trains of thought or actions at one time. This ability has benefits but also brings the challenges of becoming overly focused on rumination, worry and hyper-awareness. In addition, people may use coping strategies such as numbing via substance misuse or self-harm to deal with distressing emotions and bodily sensations.

The compassion-focused exercises provided, can be used as a more helpful or adaptive way of coping with emotions such as fear, anger, anxiety or sadness and the bodily sensations we have when experiencing these emotions.

1. Compassion-oriented goals and values: Being altruistic, helping and comforting others.
2. Soothing rhythm breathing: Breathing can be paired with a word (e.g., peace, kindness, calm, love) or a phrase (e.g., 'soften soothe allow') that becomes linked to calming breathing.
3. Loving kindness practices: 'May all people feel love and peace' can be used as a mantra in meditation.

These exercises can be combined with actions like putting one's hand on one's cheek or on one's heart area. Neuroscientific research supports the calming effects of these approaches on the body.

4. Mindfulness: Mindfulness is described as keeping your attention in the present moment without judgement. Given that our minds are prone to wander, we can make choices about what our mind focuses on. With mindfulness, we can learn to slow the busy multitasking mind down. Mindfulness can give us the chance to notice or observe a thought, feeling and/or sensation and 'be in' the moment.
5. The 4 Cs: Catch it, check it, change it with compassion:
   Catch it = Notice the thought, feeling or sensation.
   Check it = Stay with the experience without judgement.
   Change it = Shift or change the thought and cope with it using a compassionate approach. Bring compassion to the thought, feeling or experience to increase soothing and connection with self and others.
6. Body scan: Notice tightness, anxiety or fear in your body. Let go of tension in your neck, shoulders, jaw, chest or wherever you carry stress. Take a few moments throughout each day to pay attention to, and de-stress your body.
7. Imagery: Create an image of a compassionate person/being, or create imagery of a place of contentment you can go to. Use all your senses to enhance the image. Humans are visual beings, and imagery can be a powerful tool to affect how we think, feel and ultimately behave.

When creating an image of a compassionate being or nurturer, use all the senses to make the image as real as possible (looks, feels, smells, sounds and taste). Those who have interpersonal difficulties or traumas may start with an inanimate object or animal. If bringing compassion to the self is challenging, start with caring for others and then bring that compassion to yourself gradually.

8. Letter writing: Write a caring letter to yourself. Bring compassion and caring to yourself, including past and current difficult experiences and feelings.

9. Compassionate self-correction: We all have a tendency to focus on our mistakes or potential for making an error. We do have a choice in how we notice and respond to errors, bringing a compassionate self-correction approach instead of self-criticism or self-shaming. For example, from 'What an idiot I am' to 'How can I get through this and learn something from my mistakes?'

10. Compassionate attention: Use mindfulness; remember times when you have coped and others have been kind to you.

11. Compassionate thinking and reasoning: Think of what you would say to a good friend if they were experiencing a similar situation to yourself.

12. Compassionate behaviour or actions: Engage in 'random acts of kindness', take a soothing bath, act toward yourself as you would a friend or family member.

13. Compassionate sensing: Use soothing rhythmic breathing and calming smells such as lavender.

See the books and websites in the list at the end of the chapter for more detailed information and instructions for these exercises. There are guided audio exercises that you can use to do the compassion-focused exercises discussed in this chapter.

Summary of Key CFT Approaches: Dos and Don'ts

Do ... Notice self-critical thoughts and anxious, fearful and suspicious thoughts and feelings. It is important to know what you are thinking in order to figure out how to help yourself feel better.

Do ... Use a compassionate image when you are feeling fearful, anxious or down about yourself.

Do ... Practice self-compassion mindfulness. Slow your breathing, take up a relaxed position, relax your facial muscles, then focus on feelings of kindness and a desire to be caring.

Do ... Ask yourself what a compassionate other might say about something you are struggling with.

Do ... Be aware of possible barriers and work on overcoming them first.

Many of us have barriers to compassion, caring and positive emotions, for example, feelings of not deserving compassion, fears about being vulnerable, anxiousness about letting one's 'guard down', beliefs that a harsh approach to oneself or others is motivating and fears of compassion (being weak).

Don't ... Expect quick change.

Don't ... Challenge the other person in an attempt to disprove their experiences, but rather offer a compassionate ear to listen to their experiences.

Reference

Braehler, C., Harper, J., & Gilbert, P. (2013) Compassion focused group therapy for recovery after psychosis. In C. Steel (ed.), *CBT for schizophrenia: Evidence-based interventions and future directions* (pp. 235–66). Chichester, UK: Wiley.

Additional Reading

Gaudiano, B. A. (2015) *Treating depression in psychosis.* In *Incorporating acceptance and mindfulness into the treatment of psychosis: Current trends and future directions* (pp. 81–102). New York: Oxford University Press.

Germer, C. K. & Siegel, R. D. (2012) *Wisdom and compassion in psychotherapy*. New York: The Guilford Press.

Germer, C. K. (2009) *The mindful path to self-compassion: Freeing yourself from destructive thoughts and emotions*. New York: The Guilford Press.

Gilbert, P. (2009) *The compassionate mind*. London: Constable & Robinson.

(2010). *Compassion-focused therapy*. New York: Routledge.

(2014) *Mindful compassion: How the science of compassion can help you understand your emotions, live in the present, and connect deeply with others*. Oakland, CA: Constable & Robinson.

Neff, K. (2011) *Self-compassion*. New York: HarperCollins Publishers.

Tirch, D. D. & Gilbert, P. (2012) *The compassionate-mind guide to overcoming anxiety*. Oakland, CA: New Harbinger Publications, Inc.

Welford, M. (2013) *The power of self-compassion: Using compassion-focused therapy to end self-criticism and build self-confidence*. Oakland, CA: New Harbinger Publications, Inc.

Wright, N. P., Turkington, D., Kelly, O., Davies, D., Jacobs, A., & Hopton, J. (2014) *Treating psychosis: A clinician's guide to integrating acceptance and commitment therapy, compassion-focused therapy & mindfulness approaches within the cognitive behavioral therapy tradition*. Oakland, CA: New Harbinger Publications, Inc.

Websites and Other Info

www.compassionforvoices.com
www.compassionatemindco.uk

www.mindfulselfcompassion.org
www.self-compassion.org
www.mindfulcompassion.com
www.cultureofempathy.com/References/Experts/Paul-Gilbert.htm
www.intervoiceonline.org
www.amazon.com/Learning-Voices-Head-Books-Book-ebook/dp/B00ECJNSS6
www.compassionforvoices.com
TED Talk by Dr Eleanor Longden: The Voices in My Head

Links to Other Chapters

Compassion-focused approaches are woven through the chapters in the book. They can be used to reduce distress associated with stigma and trauma, including the experience of distressing beliefs, voices and visions. Compassion-focused approaches can be used to notice and address worry, rumination and avoidance. Compassion-focused approaches can be used to deal with stress and reduce triggers, catastrophic appraisals and social isolation. Compassion can influence our thinking, belief development and beliefs about the future. Through connection/affiliation and soothing, social defeat and negative symptoms can be reduced. This can then enhance drive/motivation and the ability to engage in meaningful goals. Finally, compassion-focused approaches can be used to have a powerful positive effect on the individual experiencing psychosis, their family and carers, the health care system and ultimately society.

13 Improving Self-Care, Attention/ Memory, Motivation and Social Functioning

Dawn I. Velligan, Matt Brown

Key Points

1. When we can't remember things well and keep our focus, planning ordinary activities may seem too difficult. Our motivation to do things may just not be there. Attention, memory, planning and motivation play a large role in our ability to carry out day-to-day activities.

2. Schizophrenia often leads to problems in attention, memory, planning and motivation. These problems in thinking and motivation lead to struggles with activities that involve self-care, home care, being productive during the day, socialising with others, managing finances and other common daily activities.

3. Research has demonstrated that strategies and aids can be used in someone's home or work environment to help them perform a variety of day-to-day activities. Using aids to help someone remember or plan can lessen how much a person needs to rely on their own thinking resources. These are designed to specifically help bypass problems in memory, attention and planning, and can make it easier for a person to do important tasks.

Introduction

Most of us at some time in our lives will experience an event or series of events that challenges our ability to function on a daily basis. Loss and grief are examples of this. During periods of profound grief, it is common for people to have difficulty performing everyday tasks because it becomes hard to focus one's mind and energy. In the throes of grief people often describe it being hard to think and concentrate. It can also become hard to find the motivation to do things. Individuals who are living with schizophrenia face similar challenges in thinking and motivation.

Sometimes, those dealing with the impact of schizophrenia have trouble paying attention, remembering what needs to be done, solving problems that come up or even keeping track of things. These problems in thinking can clearly make everyday activities harder to do. For example, if you have trouble planning, you may not be able to figure out when to wake up to catch a bus on time or to make it to a doctor's appointment. You may forget to do things you said you would do, thereby making others angry. You may have trouble following a long explanation or story by a doctor, parent or friend. It may also be very hard to follow new and unfamiliar instructions given by a doctor or other treatment professional.

In addition to these thinking difficulties, individuals with schizophrenia often have trouble with motivation. When we don't have motivation, it is easy to be overwhelmed by the everyday activities that other people take for granted. Troubles with motivation make it difficult to start and complete daily activities such as managing medication, bathing, cleaning your room or home, doing laundry, preparing a meal or managing finances. These activities may feel like they are too much for someone who is using their resources and energy to cope with symptoms of an illness such as schizophrenia.

For carers and friends it is important to know that problems in thinking and motivation are not signs that a person is lazy, but real symptoms of the illness. Because of this, it may be hard for carers or friends to know when and how hard to nudge someone to become more independent and engaged in the world. Research has shown that modifying a person's environment using organisational and memory aids, as well as new strategies for approaching everyday tasks, are effective tools for making activities easier and increasing motivation and success (Allott et al. 2016; Velligan et al. 2000, 2002, 2008a, 2008b).

We all use aids to help us get through our day. We have buzzers and alarms for our cars so we don't leave our keys in them. We make lists when we go shopping so we don't forget to buy something we need. We use calendars and appointment books to help us stay organised and remember appointments and meetings. We even make notes for ourselves so we don't forget things we consider important. This chapter describes how to use aids such as these to help individuals with schizophrenia experience greater success in carrying out daily activities. Table 13.1 provides a list and brief description of the various aids we cover in this chapter.

Table 13.1 List of aids to use in the living space that help with completing daily activities

Aid	Description
Signs	Should be big, bold, colourful and placed at eye level in heavily used areas to serve as memory aids and/or prompt an action. A refrigerator door or the back of the front door can serve as good locations. Changing the colour of signs can help to maintain their effectiveness.
Pill container	Provides a way to organise and track medication. Especially useful for medication schedules that are complex or involve multiple medications. Pill boxes are available for each day of the week, dividing days of the week into a.m. and p.m. compartments, and are even available to store medication for an entire month.
Alarms	Alarms provide an alert that something needs to be attended to. They can help refocus attention on a task or cue an action like taking medication.
Calendar	Calendars provide an aid for planning and scheduling activities such as appointments and serve as reminders for them. Large desk calendars hung on a wall can be easier to work with.
Daily schedules	A daily schedule can help someone keep on track with the activities they want to do over the course of their day. It provides a means of seeing what has been done and what remains to be done.
Checklists	Checklists provide step-by-step instructions for completing daily activities that reduce the effort of having to rely on one's own attention, memory and planning to complete an activity.
Audio-recorded instructions	Audio-recorded instructions serve the same purpose as checklists. They may be more helpful when someone has difficulty keeping track of what is on a list, or if a person just responds better to verbal rather than written instruction.
Organising the environment	Arranging and grouping items in someone's living space to make an activity easier to do. For example, placing a pill container on a dresser, next to a clock, with bottles of water puts what is needed to take medication together in one place. It also puts these items where they are likely to be noticed at bedtime or upon waking, common times for taking medication.

Supports can help someone who is struggling to take care of day-to-day activities. Supports like signs, lists, alarms, etc., can be set up in the home to remind someone to do important things, help someone go step by step through an activity and make everyday jobs easier to start. Using these aids, day-to-day activities can be checked off as completed, and a person can begin to experience successes in this area of their life again. Even small accomplishments or successes can make people more willing to try again. When a person is able to complete each individual step of a task that involves multiple steps, like doing laundry, ultimately he finds his clothes washed, folded and placed in the drawers or hung in the closet. The key is to find the right aids for an individual. As carers it will be important to notice and highlight all efforts to move, do and function. The completion of any one step of a task is as important as the completion of the entire task in terms of motivating further progress and effort. It is important to remember that individuals are making an effort to do an activity in the face of thinking problems and trouble with motivation. This makes each attempt a success!

Personal Disclosure

During a particularly stressful period in school, my grandmother died. It just so happens she was the person in our family I had the greatest fondness for. She was generally known as the family grump, but I adored her, and her loss hit me quite hard. After returning home from the funeral, I found it quite hard to concentrate on anything, and all the things that seemed so important before seemed trivial now. Looking back at that period of grief in my life, I can honestly say I bathed less frequently, ate fast food more often, maintained less contact with other people in my life and felt generally uninterested in doing much of anything. I was consumed by my feeling of loss. I was often distracted and would lose track of what I was doing. I remember one particular day becoming quite frustrated over having to read the same paragraph for a fifth time because I was unable to concentrate on what I was reading. For me, this period of my life provides a clear example that the things we experience in life can have a profound impact on how we function on a day-to-day basis. I consider myself fortunate that the intensity of my grief subsided and I was able to return to a regular routine. For others who have been coping with the onset of psychosis, the effects of their experiences can be similar in nature to those experienced during grief. Psychosis can have a profound impact on carrying out the day-to-day activities of living.

Have you ever experienced a time when you had a large number of important demands on your life all at once? Think back to that time. Did you notice it was more difficult to remember to do some things because you were focused on other things? Did your ability to concentrate cause you to forget what it was that you were in the middle of doing? Did simple problems seem too hard to solve? Did you feel overwhelmed and have trouble even starting to do some things? Can you describe a time in your life when you were more distracted and you found that doing everyday activities was more difficult?

Positive Aspects

What looks to observers like inactivity and lack of motivation may represent an attempt on the part of the person to protect himself or herself. Withdrawing from activities and people can be a protective response for someone who is overwhelmed by all of the information that is coming in, or who is having trouble remembering and paying attention. Hallucinations and delusions are experiences that intrude upon a person's thoughts and awareness. As such, they can consume a great deal of mental energy and take up many of the thinking resources a person needs to do daily activities. Isolation and inactivity are behaviours that might protect a person when symptoms are particularly strong. Isolation and inactivity limit exposure to things in the world that may overwhelm a person's thinking resources. To carers and others watching the person who withdraws, it may seem like an unhelpful or even unhealthy response. However, it is important to recognise that this behaviour may serve an important and beneficial purpose for an individual. Once the intensity of the psychosis subsides, sometimes people stay stuck in this protective response. It can be a healthy goal to increase an individual's activity and engagement. We can use strategies and aids to make daily activities manageable and create opportunities for success. Successful experiences demonstrate to a person that they can engage with the outside world without a high risk of becoming overwhelmed. Successes, even small ones, can be powerful experiences that increase a person's chance of doing future activities. This is especially true when someone may have been struggling to do things for a long time and it has affected their confidence. Repeated and prolonged difficulty doing everyday activities can create feelings of hopelessness. Experiences of success have the potential to combat lost confidence and feelings of hopelessness.

Simple Example

Zoey is a 24-year-old woman who has struggled with hearing voices for the past five years. She lives in a guest room behind her older sister's house. Her sister is very busy, juggling married life with three children and a full-time job. Although her sister provides support and assistance when able, Zoey is responsible for taking care of her own needs, but she has trouble remembering things. As a result, she often forgets to take her medication, sometimes misses doctor appointments, forgets to go shopping when she is getting low on food, forgets to do her laundry, etc. Zoey is fortunate that her medication does help with her symptoms, such as the voices she hears. When she forgets to take her medication, the voices are worse and she tends to feel more overwhelmed by them, making everything else more difficult. However, even when she is taking her medication, it does not help Zoey with her memory. In an effort to help, Zoey's sister gave her an appointment book to write things down so Zoey could remember things. When Zoey's sister asked her why she wasn't using the notebook, Zoey explained that she often doesn't use it because she forgets to do so. Although her sister was taking a step in the right direction and offering a reasonable solution, Zoey could likely use a bit more help with remembering things.

As shown by Zoey's example, problems with memory can affect many areas of our daily lives. A number of strategies have been shown to help with daily activities when memory is a problem. The strategies we lay out in this chapter can be implemented by individuals living with schizophrenia, their family members or other carers. We start with aids that help someone remember to take medication. These same aids can be used to help Zoey remember and do many of the other day-to-day activities she is having trouble with. We will describe these in further detail as we present the aids and how to apply them. As a first step, it is important to pick one area at a time to work on. As an individual develops success in that one area, make sure to take time with them to discuss what it feels like for them to have achieved this success. For Zoey, she was feeling disheartened by repeatedly forgetting to take care of things. This affected her confidence in herself, and she began to view herself as less capable. Zoey's reaction is not unusual. This is the kind of response many people have when they find themselves struggling to complete daily activities such as caring for one's self and home. For this and other reasons, it is important to take time with a person to help them acknowledge and experience their own success. Once someone has consistently demonstrated success in one area with the use of these aids, they can be used in other areas.

Taking Medication

Although there are a number of reasons someone may not take their medication, Zoey is willing to take her medications and believes they help her. Because she often forgets to take her medication, this is a good area to apply environmental aids to help Zoey. Most of us, at one time or another, have tried to take daily medication such as antibiotics or even daily vitamins. Even without memory problems, most people have experienced that moment where they cannot remember if they took their medication. Sometimes people get distracted on the way to the kitchen by their phone ringing and don't remember if they took it. The difficulty of remembering to take medication or remembering whether medication was taken is increased greatly when multiple medications are involved that need to be taken at different times a day, when the dosage of a medication changes depending on the time of day or when different medications are supposed to be taken under different conditions. For example, one medication is supposed to be taken on an empty stomach and another medication with meals.

Signs

Posting signs for Zoey can provide visual reminders and prompts for her to take her medication. Signs can reduce the need for Zoey to rely on her memory by providing the information she is having trouble remembering right where she can see, in her living space. Signs are most effective in frequently trafficked locations, such as the back of a front door or on a refrigerator door. The most effective location will depend on an individual's daily routine. If the person does not leave their house often, then a sign on the front door will have little benefit. Similarly, if someone does not go into the kitchen very often, then a sign on the refrigerator is not very helpful. What we know about Zoey is that each morning she will make a bowl of cereal for herself in the kitchen. This means she opens the refrigerator to get the milk. She also likes to snack during the day, usually on baby carrots and grapes, both of which she keeps in the refrigerator. This means that in the morning and other times throughout an average day, Zoey will open the refrigerator. Posting a sign on the refrigerator door would be a good choice because she is going to come into contact with it repeatedly during the day. It is also helpful to place the same sign at different locations to increase the chances that Zoey will come in contact with it during the course of her day. We know that Zoey will often go outside to sit in her sister's yard, which means that the front door would also be a good place for a sign so that she sees it when she goes outside. Signs should be simple, on brightly coloured paper, easy to read and placed at eye level in order to be the most effective. By changing the colour of these signs every week, they will continue to capture Zoey's attention and be more likely to lead to her taking medication at all dosing times.

Example Sign

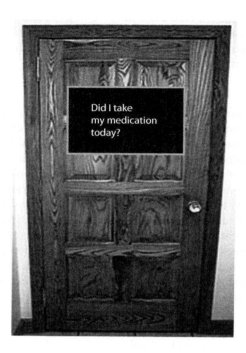

Did I take
my medication
today?

Pill Container to Aid Organisation

The use of a pill container may be a helpful aid for Zoey in a number of different ways. Pill containers can be placed in plain view as a cue to take medication. This reduces reliance on memory. Filling a medication container once a week can provide an alert for Zoey that she will run out of her medication soon, prompting her to refill her prescriptions. The container also provides a way for her to see whether or not she has taken her medication at a specific time. For example, if Wednesday morning's medication is still in the compartment at lunch time, she can easily see that she did not take her morning medication. Zoey does not need to make an effort to try to remember if she did or did not take her medication that morning. All she has to do is look inside her pill container, and if there are more pills left in a compartment than there should be, she knows she did not take her medication for that dosing time.

The first step to setting up a pill container is to find the right container. The right container will be one that is easy to organise, simple to use and will store medication for all dosing times. If she only takes one medication once a day, a simple seven-day pill box with compartments to hold medication for each day may be fine.

If Zoey takes medication more than once per day, a seven-day pill box with separate a.m. and p.m. compartments for each day may be better. This would be especially helpful

Lids closed – days of the week

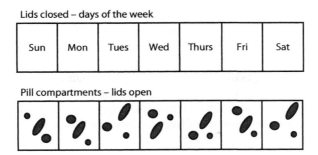

Sun	Mon	Tues	Wed	Thurs	Fri	Sat

Pill compartments – lids open

if Zoey is taking different medications in the morning and evening. The separate a.m./ p.m. compartments can be particularly helpful for separating and organising medications to be taken at different times of the day. A large variety of different pill boxes are available to suit the various needs individuals may have.

Lids closed – days of the week with a compartment for the morning, and for the evening

Sun AM	Mon AM	Tues AM	Wed AM	Thurs AM	Fri AM	Sat AM
Sun PM	Mon PM	Tues PM	Wed PM	Thurs PM	Fri PM	Sat PM

Pill compartments – lids open

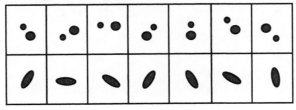

The best way a pill box can be used to help Zoey remember to take medication is to place it in a location that has the best chance of being seen when it is time for her to take medication. If Zoey only takes medication before bed, good places to put a pill box depend on her routine before bed. What we know for Zoey is that she brushes her teeth every night before bed. She has always done this, and it has become so automatic for her that she very rarely forgets to do it. A good place to put the pill box for Zoey may be on the shelf above the bathroom sink where she will see it when she brushes her teeth. Other people may have different routines. Knowing a person's routine is helpful for family members and carers to find the best location to put an aid like a pill box.

Several simple questions can be helpful. Does she set an alarm or check the clock before bed? Does she use the bathroom to brush her teeth or wash her face before bed? Does she watch TV in her room before going to sleep? Placing a pill container in a location where Zoey regularly interacts often gives it the best chance to remind her to take her medication. In the picture below, medication and water bottles (to make taking medication easier) are placed right on the nightstand of the bed. This way they can be seen before going to sleep. No additional steps such as going to the kitchen for water are required. By decreasing the number of steps to complete this task, it is more likely that the person will do it.

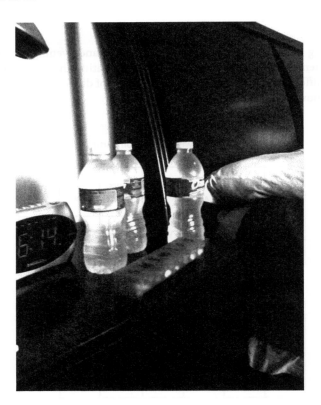

Using an Alarm Clock

Alarms are an important tool that may often be overlooked. Some people tend to respond better to visual cues like signs, but other people respond better to sound cues. When we think of alarms, alarm clocks often come to mind. However, kitchen timers, microwaves, small pocket timers and handheld devices can also be used to provide an alarm as a reminder or attention getter. For Zoey, an alarm is an added tool to help her remember. Providing multiple reminders through different formats gives the best chance to help Zoey remember to take her medication. Setting an alarm that she knows indicates it is time to take her medication, further reduces Zoey's need to rely on memory.

Alarm clocks with features such as voice recording can be very helpful. A person can then hear the message in their own words (e.g., 'It's 8 a.m. Time to take my medication' or 'I want to take medication so I can take some classes'). Devices that allow you to set multiple alarms are especially useful for helping someone remember to take medication at different times of the day. These alarms can also be used to prompt other activities like waking up, time for exercise, time to feed animals and other important daily routines. Medication alarm clock apps are also available for mobile devices such as smart phones. Using a smart phone may be helpful because they are usually kept with the owner. It is important not to overwhelm someone with too many different alarms during the day. It is best to start simple, with the one target like remembering to take medication, and see how someone responds to the use of the alarm. If someone finds it effective and helpful, other alarm messages may be added.

Before we move on to help Zoey with other daily activities, we want to take some time to find out how it feels for her to successfully take her medication. Does she realise this is something that she is now doing that she was having trouble with before? How does that feel for her? What does this mean about other areas she may be having trouble with? Does this mean that maybe these same kinds of aids can help her in other areas?

Calendars and Daily Schedules

Similar to the appointment book Zoey's sister got her, calendars and daily schedules can be very helpful for someone who forgets appointments. Large calendars and schedules have an advantage over appointment books because they can be placed on a door, refrigerator or wall in plain sight to increase the chances they will be used. An appointment book may not help if it is left on a desk top or in a purse. It may simply go unnoticed or be forgotten. Placing tools such as calendars and schedules in the sight line of someone during their daily routine is what makes them effective tools for aiding memory. A calendar can be filled out at the beginning of each month or week to track important dates and appointments. A desktop-sized calendar hung on a door, wall or refrigerator is large enough to grab attention and easier to write on. Note that it is good to always attach a pen or marker to it so that the calendar will be used. If someone has to search for something to write with, this decreases the likelihood that the person will use the calendar. Zoey could learn the habit of checking her calendar the night before or in the morning to see if she has any appointments or other plans she needs to pay attention to and plan for.

Although many calendars are used to show weekly or monthly schedules, a daily activity schedule can be used to help Zoey remember the activities she needs to do over the course of a day. It can serve as a reminder to check her calendar for appointments that day. It can also prompt important daily behaviours she may be overlooking. A personalised list of activities like the one below may be helpful.

Helping Zoey

When we began telling Zoey's story, we mentioned that her memory was interfering with her taking her medicine, keeping doctor appointments, doing her laundry and shopping for food. We listed a number of aids that can help Zoey remember each of these activities, not just remembering to take her medication. Signs, alarms, calendars and schedules can be used to help Zoey remember any or all of these activities each day. The pill container is

Things I did today

Check the box for each activity you do during the day

Activity	Monday	Tuesday	Wednesday	Thursday	Friday	Saturday	Sunday
Took my medicine							
Took a shower or bath							
Brushed my teeth							
Changed my clothes							
Made a meal							
Got together with a friend							
Washed my clothes							

only used as an aid to remember and organise medication, but the other aids may be used to help in many areas of a person's life. It's what makes these tools so effective. They can be adapted to many different situations and set up for a specific person's needs.

More Complex Example

Jeremy is a 33-year-old man who has been living with the effects of schizophrenia for the past 16 years. He lives alone in an apartment with the help of a housing assistance programme. He spends most of his day watching TV or listening to music. He spends so much of his time in idle activities because he has trouble completing many daily activities. Similar to Zoey, Jeremy has difficulty with memory, but he also struggles with keeping his attention focused on things as well as organising and planning out how to do activities. Like Zoey, he also has trouble keeping his doctor appointments. However, he doesn't just forget them sometimes. Jeremy also struggles to figure out how to take the bus to get there. It is hard for him to plan how long the trip will take and when to leave. He also has a hard time figuring out which buses to take to get to the clinic. He is having similar problems with activities like bathing, doing his laundry, cooking and cleaning his apartment. Even when he begins one of these activities, he finds it hard to concentrate on them and will often leave them unfinished. Jeremy regularly feels bad about not doing these things. It has been a repeated source of conflict between him and his mother. When his mother visits, she often becomes upset over the state of her son and his living environment. She repeatedly tells Jeremy that he needs to take better care of himself and that she doesn't understand why he won't at least just clean the place up. Jeremy's mother is not unique in expressing such concerns, but she may be unaware of how truly overwhelming these kinds of activities feel for Jeremy. Jeremy may have no idea where to start. It also may be very hard for him to explain to his mother why these things are so hard for him.

Although these tasks may seem ordinary, Jeremy is faced with serious challenges in doing them. Laundry provides a good example because it is an ordinary, everyday task that uses all three areas of thinking that Jeremy is struggling with. Completing a load of laundry requires doing a series of steps in a specific order. This means he needs to be able to think through and plan out the steps he needs to complete. He also needs to be able to keep track of which step he is on, what materials are needed, which steps he has completed and which step is next. Being able to do this requires him to use his memory and stay focused on what he is doing. Otherwise, he may forget detergent after he has already walked to the laundry room, he may leave wet clothing in the washer to sour or he may leave dry clothing in the laundry room. Jeremy needs to be able to remember and pay attention to all the details he needs to successfully do his laundry. These could include things like making sure to bring all the needed supplies, adding the right amount of detergent, bringing enough money to use a pay machine and not leaving laundry in the washer overnight. So, the everyday task of doing laundry requires using three areas of thinking, including planning and organising, paying attention and remembering. Imagine for a moment how difficult doing a load of laundry could be if you were having problems in all these areas. Doing laundry is made even harder for Jeremy because of his problems with organising and planning, which has led to a heaped pile of clean and dirty clothes mixed together on the closet floor. Before he even begins laundry, he faces the challenge of figuring out a plan for dealing with this pile of clothes. Does he just wash them all even though some are not dirty? What if he doesn't have enough money to wash them all? How does he tell dirty clothes from clean? How does he separate them, and where does he put them? How is he going to keep track of what he is doing and remember which pile is which? Faced with these challenges, Jeremy sometimes feels overwhelmed just walking into his room to get his clothes for laundry and gives up on it.

Let's discuss what Jeremy and his mother can do to make activities like laundry, cleaning and getting to a doctor's office easier for him. In order to help Jeremy, we need to provide aids that will help with all three of the areas he is having trouble with: memory, attention and planning.

All of the aids we talked about for helping Zoey could also be used for Jeremy, including a pill container, signs, using alarms, a calendar and a daily schedule. We need to add a couple new strategies to help Jeremy because he is also having trouble with his attention and planning how to do things. We want to make sure that aids like signs can be effective for someone who is having a hard time focusing their attention. We want to make sure signs stand out and grab his attention. Bigger, bolder and more colourful signs are a good strategy to use in order to draw his attention to them. The sign below on the left does not stand out and grab attention. The sign on the right does.

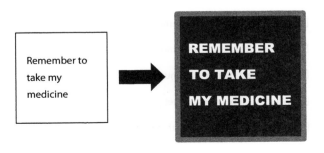

Placing signs in more locations also increases the chance they get his attention. We need to be careful, though. We only want to use enough aids to help Jeremy do his activities. His trouble with attention and planning means that too many different aids or signs about different things would not be helpful for him. They would be more likely to overwhelm him. We want to pick only the aids and strategies that will work best for him. For example, we may not use both a daily schedule and calendar for Jeremy because this may be too much information at once. We'll start with a calendar to simply help him remember appointments in the beginning. As he learns to use an aid and becomes more comfortable with it, we can add something new like a daily schedule, but only if adding it is helpful.

Checklists

Another important tool to help with memory, especially when someone is having trouble keeping focused on what they are doing, is to put together a checklist with each step of a task. A checklist provides step-by-step instructions for doing a task. It also provides Jeremy a way to keep track of doing his laundry by putting a check mark next to the step he just finished. Both of these aspects of checklists will be helpful for Jeremy by allowing him to rely less on his own memory, concentration and planning to finish his laundry. Checklists should be simple, straightforward and easy to follow. Therefore, the checklist should be made up of the fewest steps that make sense to finish an activity. An example checklist for doing laundry is presented below.

LAUNDRY CHECKLIST
Grab a pen or pencil!
AFTER YOU FINISH EACH STEP CHECK THE BOX NEXT TO IT

☐ Get your laundry basket, detergent, a pencil, and laundry money.

☐ Put the clothes you want to wash from laundry hamper in your basket

☐ Take your laundry, detergent, and money to the washing machine.

☐ Put your clothes into the machine and add detergent.

☐ Set temperature to warm or cold.

☐ Close washing machine lid and start the machine.

☐ Set your pocket timer to go off in 30 minutes and clip it to your pocket.

☐ Leave this checklist on the washer.

☐ When the timer goes off remove clothes from washer and place in dryer.

☐ Choose heat setting and start dryer.

☐ Set pocket timer for 40 minutes and clip it to your pocket.

☐ When the timer goes off, get your clothes from the dryer.

☐ Fold your clothes and put them in the drawer they belong in.

Audio-Recorded Instructions

To help him keep on track with doing his laundry, we have provided Jeremy a checklist of step-by-step instructions. The benefit of written instructions can sometimes vary and may be limited by Jeremy's trouble keeping his attention focused. If Jeremy is having enough trouble with attention, it may be difficult for him to follow along through a list of step-by-step instructions written out on a sheet of paper. In this case, an audio recording of the step-by-step instructions in real time may be helpful. Audio recordings are easy tools for an individual to use and may be made for any task that requires a series of smaller steps to complete. Even bathing or brushing teeth can be broken down into smaller steps. Step-by-step instructions, either with a checklist or audio recording, can be provided for as many different activities as is helpful for someone.

Using Alarms

Faced with both memory and attention problems, there's a fair chance that after his laundry is in the machine and ready to be put into the dryer, Jeremy will have forgotten about it. His attention is easily drawn away from things, which makes it harder for him to keep track of what he is doing. An audio alarm is a particularly helpful aid to grab his attention and alert him there is something he needs to do. For something like laundry, a pocket timer that he can carry with him is ideal. Set to go off in 30 minutes after he starts the wash, it will provide a cue for Jeremy that his laundry needs to be moved from the washer to the dryer. Instructions to set the timer and what to do when the timer goes off are specified on the checklist. Instructions may include leaving the checklist on the washer to reduce the chance it will be misplaced.

Strategically Arranging the Living Space

Another way we can help Jeremy do his laundry is to help him organise his clothes in a way that makes separating clean and dirty clothes easier and makes it easier for him to store his clothes. A simple laundry hamper placed right next to where Jeremy removes his clothing can be helpful. Hampers and baskets are less helpful if they are in a closet where they will not be seen and are a distance away from where Jeremy undresses. A coloured sign with big bold letters on the hamper saying 'DIRTY CLOTHES GO HERE' and signs on each drawer of the dresser can help Jeremy keep dirty and clean clothes separate. This makes it easier to get his dirty clothes ready for laundry and to put them away when he has finished.

Arranging someone's living space to make doing an activity easier can be applied to many activities. Jeremy is also having trouble keeping his apartment clean. When we ask about his cleaning supplies, we find that they are scattered through various areas of his apartment in different rooms and cabinets. The various cleaning tools and supplies he needs to use are not easily accessible and organised for ease of use. In order to clean, Jeremy has to start with remembering which supplies are left where. The difficulty of being able to remember this information reduces the chances that he will make it to the step where he begins to clean. One simple aid would be to provide a cleaning tote where he can have all of his supplies stored together so that they may be carried around easily to any place in his apartment he would like to clean. This is a simple organising tool that groups everything needed for an activity together. It reduces the need for someone to rely on their ability to remember, plan and maintain focus to complete an activity. It allows for a more grab-and-go approach.

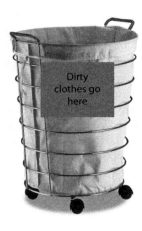

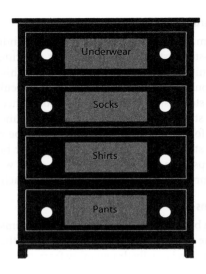

Helping Jeremy

As we have discussed, Jeremy is having trouble with a number of day-to-day activities. Now that we have put in place a number of aids that will help him to do his laundry, we need to think about how we can use these same tools to help him with his other activities. We discussed how we can organise his cleaning supplies to make it easier for him to clean his home. We can also add a checklist or audio-recorded instructions for general cleaning, or cleaning specific areas (e.g., the kitchen or bathroom) if needed. How might we use these aids to help Jeremy take the bus so he makes his doctor appointments? We could make a checklist for him that includes how long it takes to make the trip, what buses to take, when to switch buses, where to get on the buses and where to get off. We can also provide Jeremy with a bus schedule including instructions and practice with using it to figure out when to start a 45-minute bus trip to get to the clinic.

All of the tools we have presented in the examples for Zoey and Jeremy are adaptable. They can be tailored to individuals and different activities. You may not find the right aid or set of aids that are helpful for someone on the first attempt. It may take tinkering and talking about what is helpful and working and what is not. Finding out how to change things so they may be more effective is part of working with these aids. Do not be discouraged if one sign placed in the hallway doesn't do the trick. Try bigger signs with bright colours, add an alarm too or place the sign in a different location based on the person's daily habits.

Lastly, it is worth re-emphasising the importance of taking time to help someone recognise and experience their successes. For most people who are living with the effects of schizophrenia, daily activities can be difficult. Some people have experienced what they view as repeated failures in taking care of things. This can feed the belief that they are not capable and act against the motivation to even attempt activities. For someone who has experienced this, making an effort to do an activity can be viewed as an exercise in courage and perseverance. Even the attempt itself may be a success for someone who has stopped attempting. When someone has success completing an activity or part of an activity with the use of an aid, that success needs to be recognised and experienced. This is especially important because it reinforces the belief that someone can do activities they thought they could not do. It makes explicit the benefit of these tools, and that may increase someone's commitment to using them. Discussing how an activity like laundry has made things better for someone, connects their success to real benefits. Maybe their clothes don't smell anymore and this has affected the way others act around them. Maybe it just feels good to know they are wearing clean clothes. Most important, experiencing success is an excellent motivator for wanting to try again or try something new.

Summary of Key Techniques

- Environmental cues such as signs or alarms can be used as memory aids and to prompt initiation of an activity such as bathing or taking medication. Signs should be easy to read and easy to see. A variety of alarms can also be used to cue memory or grab attention, including clocks, cooking timers, microwaves and handheld electronic devices like smart phones.
- Pill containers can be used to help organise medication, as a cue for taking medication and as a check for whether medication was taken. A large variety of containers are available to meet individual needs.
- Checklists and audio-recorded instructions are helpful aids for any activity that can be broken down into individual steps to complete in order. These aids are helpful for individuals having difficulty in any area of thinking, including memory, attention and planning.
- Calendars and daily schedules are useful for helping someone keep appointments, plan out activities and keep track of activities when they are completed. They help people remember activities and organise them to reduce the burden of someone having to plan things out in their head.
- For someone who is having trouble with organising and planning, their living space can be organised to make tasks easier. For example, placing a hamper near the dresser so it is easier to keep clean and dirty clothes separate can make it easier to do laundry. Organising someone's living space works by making tasks easier and removing barriers that have been getting in the way of doing those tasks.
- Change it up! Change the colour of signs and checklists weekly to continue to capture attention.
- Remember to help someone acknowledge and experience each success they have had.

References

Allott, K. A., Killackey, E., Sun, P., Brewer, W. J., & Velligan, D. I. (2016) Feasibility and acceptability of cognitive adaptation training for first-episode psychosis. *Early Intervention in Psychiatry*, 10(6), 476–84. doi:10.1111/eip.12207

Velligan, D. I., Bow-Thomas, C. C., Huntzinger, C., Ritch, J., Ledbetter, N., Prihoda, T. J., & Miller, A. L. (2000) Randomized controlled trial of the use of compensatory strategies to enhance adaptive functioning in outpatients with schizophrenia. *The American Journal of Psychiatry*, 157(8), 1317–23. doi:10.1176/appi.ajp.157.8.1317 [doi]

Velligan, D. I., Prihoda, T. J., Ritch, J. L., Maples, N., Bow-Thomas, C. C., & Dassori, A. (2002) A randomized single-blind pilot study of compensatory strategies in schizophrenia outpatients. *Schizophrenia Bulletin*, 28(2), 283–92.

Velligan, D. I., Diamond, P. M., Maples, N. J., Mintz, J., Li, X., Glahn, D. C., & Miller, A. L. (2008a) Comparing the efficacy of interventions that use environmental supports to improve outcomes in patients with schizophrenia. *Schizophrenia Research*, 102(1–3), 312–19. doi:10.1016/j.schres.2008.02.005 [doi]

Velligan, D. I., Diamond, P. M., Mintz, J., et al. (2008b) The use of individually tailored environmental supports to improve medication adherence and outcomes in schizophrenia. *Schizophrenia Bulletin*, 34(3), 483–93. doi:sbm111 [pii]

Further Readings

Velligan, D. I., Prihoda, T. J., Ritch, J. L., Maples, N., Bow-Thomas, C. C., & Dassori, A. (2002) A randomized single-blind pilot study of compensatory strategies in schizophrenia outpatients. *Schizophrenia Bulletin*, 28(2), 283–92.

Websites and Other Helpful Information

An electronic version of the Cognitive Adaptation Training (CAT) manual for professionals can be obtained by contacting Matt Brown through email at brownma@uthscsa.edu.

Where Can We Learn More?

Robert Reiser, Jeremy Pelton, Nazneen Rustom

Key Points

1. Carer and family experiences with psychosis can be extremely challenging, confusing and highly stressful.
2. Mental health systems may not be particularly engaging or friendly toward families; mental health providers may be not be properly trained to help families.
3. Additional resources and vital supports are available for families and carers.
4. There is a need to be proactive and advocate for family-friendly services and effective treatment locally.

Introduction

Throughout this book, you have learned about CBT-informed caring techniques for psychosis at a basic and introductory level. Naturally, many of you will be interested in broadening the scope of your knowledge and locating additional helpful resources for support and guidance. In this chapter we aim to present information to assist family caregivers in developing helpful relationships with a service user, to identify caregiver training options and to provide additional resources for support and guidance.

Maintaining Helpful Relationships with Your Family Member

Societal stigma toward psychosis has perpetuated the idea that those who suffer from psychosis seldom recover, and this entails a demoralising and pessimistic message that often leads to further helplessness and hopelessness. Readers should now be familiar with the idea that recovery looks very different for each individual and that there is a great deal of variation between individuals' in terms of social and functional recovery. The same principle applies to families where there is a wide range of experience in terms of being able to manage relationships successfully with family members who are often chronically ill. For example, building up and improving a relationship with a family member with a medication-resistant psychosis requires significant effort, persistence, social support and skilful management. Maintaining positive relationships can be even more challenging and stressful when family members do not have insight into their illness or believe that they are not ill and don't need medication. They may be angry, suspicious and even blame other family members for their problems. Sometimes these stressful interactions can cause a vicious cycle, arousing negative emotions, perpetuating problems and making it difficult to engage together in collaborative problem solving. Because this disorder most often presents as a chronic illness with ups and downs, there is a need for families to take a long-term perspective ('running a marathon' vs. 'a sprint') and balance the need to manage crises and problems with ongoing self-care.

We believe that the same pessimistic stigmatising message noted earlier about individual's with a psychotic disorder also applies to beliefs about families' ability to be resilient and cope with these difficulties. Stigmatising beliefs held by mental health providers about families can lead to similar problems in terms of excessive pessimism and demoralisation. There is a highly regrettable history with mental health services where families were blamed for their children's serious mental illnesses. Families with long memories will recall this and feel rightfully indignant and even suspicious or sceptical about services. Yet families are the ultimate safety net for people who are chronically ill – when services are not available or are restricted, we look to families to fill in the gaps.

A complicating factor in improving this picture is the fact that resources are not readily available to families (we will note exceptions to this rule in the final section of this chapter), and the mental health system is often not friendly or encouraging to families. Unfortunately, systemic shortcomings in access to physical and mental health care are often rooted in social stigma:

> The negative impact of public stigma is also observed in the general health care system; people labeled mentally ill are less likely to benefit from the depth and breadth of available physical health care services than people without these illnesses.
>
> (Corrigan & Phelan, 2004)

In addition, mental health providers often lack the proper training to provide effective family-focused care and may be philosophically predisposed to individually oriented treatment. In some cases, families can be shut out of care and excluded from participating at all, despite compelling evidence that family involvement is quite critical to good outcomes. At times, privacy rules ('Health Insurance Portability and Accountability Act (HIPAA)' in the United States) can be used as a shield to inappropriately exclude families completely from care. We argue that there is a moral imperative to include families wherever possible, as data from a recent study suggest the protective effect of family involvement in potentially reducing mortality rates (Kane et al. 2015). A recent study that determined mortality rates in first episode psychosis were 24x that of peers indicating the urgent need for improving patient and family care in psychosis (Schoenbaum et al. 2017).

One of our goals in this section is to summarise some of the research evidence and identify helpful resources relevant to building a good alliance with people who have a psychotic disorder and to develop some main principles that might help families cope more effectively in terms of improving relationships and communication with loved ones. What are some major principles to keep in mind that would lead to effective strategies when trying to develop or build up a positive, engaging relationship with a family member with psychosis? To approach the answer to this question, we look to the evidence for what is known about developing positive relationships (sometimes called 'the therapeutic alliance') in schizophrenia treatment research and how certain communication styles might be especially helpful.

We would like to mention a recent example that demonstrates how an alliance can be used to help sort out problems in a pop-culture context. In the film, *Alice Through the Looking Glass*, a sequel to Lewis Carroll's *Alice in Wonderland*, the story centres on the

Mad Hatter's seemingly delusional belief that his family is alive; when in fact, even his ally Alice is convinced that the Mad Hatter's family had passed years ago during a tragic event. The entire film is reminiscent of how a therapist might help their patient make sense of a confusing history – in this case, by developing a narrative or timeline of the events that have led the Mad Hatter to his seemingly delusional belief. While Alice attempts to examine the evidence around the seemingly delusional belief, the Mad Hatter's health deteriorates dramatically and he isolates himself. What promotes the Mad Hatter's recovery in the end, and what literally brings him *back to life*, is that fact that Alice discovered that the Mad Hatter's beliefs were grounded in real-life observation and she was able to make sense of his delusion. In some ways, this resembles the kind of approach in CBT for psychosis (CBTp) that a therapist might take to make a patient's delusions more understandable. We bring this film to your attention to simply illustrate how powerful it can be when a therapeutic connection or alliance can be formed that tries to make sense of psychosis. 'I believe you' were the key words that Alice used to bring the Mad Hatter *back to life*. Through kindness, compassion and the confidence to learn and challenge her own beliefs, Alice took the time and effort to reach within herself and to use available resources so that she could revive the Mad Hatter.

All sufferers of psychosis need an Alice. All service users need family support, or peer support or a team of professionals who have the patience to provide continuity as a witness to the often non-linear progress and setbacks that shape the world of people with psychosis. Service users need allies to venture together with them and validate the elements of underlying truth that are likely to underpin and sustain their delusional systems. How can we be more like Alice? More practically, what strategies and behaviours can we learn that can help people with psychosis?

Family Members Need Support to Care

Families can have a positive impact on members with a psychotic disorder by increasing overall warmth and support and trying to reduce conflict and stressful interactions. Let's start with discussing the value of a therapeutic alliance, or positive relationship, in CBTp. The therapeutic alliance has consistently been demonstrated to be an important predictor of improvement in psychotherapy in general (Norcross & Wampold, 2011). What exactly is the therapeutic alliance, sometimes called the helping alliance? Bordin (1979) described the alliance as composed of three elements: (1) a collaborative agreement about the goals of therapy; (2) a consensus on the tasks of therapy – what the patient must do to get better; and (3) a sense of a deep bond between the therapist and patient. How is this discussion of the therapeutic alliance relevant to carers? These main principles of collaboration, trying to agree on important goals and having a deep emotional bond, can be readily applied to non-professional helping relationships outside of therapy, that is, for caregivers and other family members interested in improving communication and relationships.

In addition to the key idea of building up a positive collaborative relationship with the service user, which is central to good CBT-informed practice, there are other good practical resources for important techniques in maintaining a positive relationship with people with psychosis. One resource includes a *Befriending Manual*, which helps caregivers steer away from distressing topics and focus on more neutral topics of mutual interest (sports, movies, books, etc.). Befriending as described in this manual (see Chapter 7) has proven to be a helpful intervention which reduces distress with certain symptoms and can improve quality of life.

Other useful principles can be drawn from the literature on *motivational interviewing*, a counselling approach that emphasises collaboration and avoiding direct arguments or disputation where you get into a position of trying to convince the other person that you are right. This often leads to a hardening of positions and engenders resistance in the other person, making them less willing to change or consider your viewpoint. One of the principles of motivational interviewing is to 'roll with the resistance' rather than getting into a confrontation or pressing your point. In general, this is consistent with CBT approaches that tend to take a gentle, inquiring and non-confrontational approach to discussing symptoms and problems.

Finally, many families have found the book by Xavier Amador, *I Am Not sick, I Don't Need Help!* to be quite valuable in terms of a communication model (LEAP: Listen, Agree, Empathise, Partner) that reduces conflict, especially when individuals lack insight into their illness and do not believe that they need medication or treatment.

Please see the end of this chapter for a summary of key take-away points.

Caregiver Training Models

Caregivers have a vitally important role to play in the social support network of a service user. Social support is a key factor associated with better outcomes across many types of mental health problems. However, the mental health system has been slow to recognise the importance of families. Research over nearly five decades determined the specific benefits that caregivers have on the service user in psychosis. Nearly 30 years ago, it was determined that a very brief four-session psychoeducation intervention could increase perceived knowledge, and furthermore reduce perceived family burden at six-month follow-up (Smith & Birchwood, 1987). Increasing knowledge of psychosis is a common component of all effective interventions for families.

Professional interventions with caregivers typically involve psychoeducation about the illness, helping manage problem behaviours, setting realistic expectations and helping to manage problem behaviours and providing emotional support. CBT-informed caring is based on the principle that caregivers can provide important long-term benefits to service users, improving quality of life and functional recovery. Programmes that have included a family psychoeducational component are known to benefit a service user's functioning and reduce hallucinations and delusions, 12 months post-intervention (Barrowclough et al. 2001). Other studies have demonstrated that families undergoing an intervention that shares CBT-like concepts that involved the family, showed long-term benefit on measures of caregiver wellbeing two years post-intervention (Addington et al. 2005; Lowenstein et al. 2010).

A key factor that is associated with relapse in psychosis is caregiver expressed emotion. Expressed emotion consists of hostile criticism or emotional overinvolvement (characterised by an overprotective, self-sacrificing style). Expressed emotion has also been shown to be an independent predictor of caregiver distress (Jansen et al. 2015) and is strongly linked to perceived psychological stress of the caregiver (Sadath et al. 2017). Caregivers low in expressed emotion are likely to reduce or delay relapse in a service user (Hogarty et al. 1986). As noted earlier there are important resources to assist families in providing a warm, supportive environment even when dealing with difficult problems.

Families can play a vital role in promoting recovery of the service user if they are empowered with solid, educational, evidence-based information. We have provided a number of useful resources, including books, websites and support groups, that are available for family carers.

A Family Member Vignette

My long journey into the world of mental illness began when my son Jake was 19 years old. At that time I had never heard of the psychiatric term 'anosognosia', which means a lack of insight into one's illness. Fifteen years later after so much frustration, anger and agony I was intimately aware of what it was like to deal with a loved one suffering from a serious mental illness who shows a lack of insight as one of their primary symptoms of the disease. This symptom of my son's schizophrenia was by far the most difficult to deal with.

I am a logical and scientific kind of person and could not understand at all how someone whose behaviour was more and more bizarre could not be made aware that there was something wrong. Jake's schizophrenia was not at all obvious for the first 10 years. He did not have either auditory or visual hallucinations but exhibited what became severe paranoia as the years passed. His symptoms also included a severe lack of motivation to do anything, obvious depression, an inability to experience pleasure, an almost complete lack of social skills and a strong tendency for self-isolation. Because he insisted that there was nothing wrong with him, which is what I wanted to believe, he was not evaluated or treated for years. In fact, I tried to give him what he said he wanted and chose to stay out of the county mental health system. My attempts at trying to convince Jake to accept help were met with angry outbursts and verbal abuse.

When his behaviour continued to deteriorate to the point that I was concerned for his safety, and my own, I had reached such a level of emotional exhaustion that I threw in the towel and, following the advice of a therapist, I contacted the National Alliance on Mental Illness (NAMI) and then the Outreach and Engagement team of the county mental health department. A trained professional member of this team specialising in anosognosia attempted to make contact with my son and talked to him several times through a closed door. Often she was met with the same kind of verbal abuse directed at me. She was an invaluable support to me and eventually encouraged me to participate in forcibly hospitalising my son with the use of the police. I could not have done this without her support. My son was hospitalised, diagnosed and treated with anti-psychotic medication for over three months. I was attending a support group for relatives of the severely mentally ill before the hospitalisation and continue to this day. Talking to other family members who experience the devastating symptoms of severe mental illness, including lack of insight, is invaluable for my own wellbeing. Learning what works in communicating with someone who does not share my reality is a skill I continue to practice with Jake. Sharing the disappointment, anger, guilt and finally intense grief in the face of an adult child with schizophrenia is now an essential part of my own healing.

Caregiver Training Programmes

Dr Douglas Turkington and his team have developed a pilot caregiver training programme in Ontario, Canada, in partnership with the Schizophrenia Society of Ontario. The objective of the training is to teach CBT-informed techniques to caregivers in a way that empowers them with knowledge, information and CBT-like methods of inquiry to understand their affected relative's psychosis. The training involves demonstrations, role-plays and direct coaching of family members (intensive model). This training aims to promote a sense of validation and self-efficacy in caregivers who often feel inadequate to help the service user and aims at developing increased knowledge of psychosis, increased sense of support and resources available and decreased helplessness.

Summary of Key Communication Strategies for Caregivers – The Dos and Don'ts

- Do ... more listening and less talking. Try to be genuinely curious about what the person with psychosis is concerned about, their worries, their personal goals and their understanding of their illness.
- Do ... try to distinguish between the symptoms of the illness and 'bad behaviour'. What looks like 'laziness' may, in fact, be part of the negative symptoms of the illness.
- Do ... try to limit giving advice and suggestions at least until the person seems ready to accept them.
- If things get heated up, it's best to turn towards a more neutral topic or take a 'let's agree to disagree' stance. Arguing a point is rarely helpful or effective and can worsen problems.
- Sometimes just shifting away from 'hot' topics (delusions, voices) to neutral topics of interest (sports, movies, books) can be quite helpful.
- Do ... try to keep the emotional 'temperature' low in all family discussions. If things get too heated, allow a cooling-off period before trying to address 'hot' issues.
- Communication with a collaborative tone is more likely to be helpful, that is, 'How can we figure things out together that would be helpful?' vs. 'You need to do X'.
- Setting goals or agreeing to tasks when there is basic agreement and where the service user sees an important personal goal or value being addressed is likely to promote engagement and 'buy-in'.
- Goals that can be broken into smaller pieces may be best. Big global goals can be overwhelming and lead to demoralisation and paralysis. Trying to break things down into smaller manageable steps can lead to a more productive approach with helpful signposts along the way.

References

Addington, J., Collins, A., McCleery, A., & Addington, D. (2005) The role of family work in early psychosis. *Schizophrenia Research*, 79(1), 77–83. doi:S0920-9964(05)00054-X [pii]

Barrowclough, C., Haddock, G., Tarrier, N., et al. (2001) Randomized controlled trial of motivational interviewing, cognitive behavior therapy, and family intervention for patients with comorbid schizophrenia and substance use disorders. *The American Journal of Psychiatry*, 158(10), 1706–13. doi:10.1176/appi.ajp.158.10.1706 [doi]

Bordin, E. S. (1979) The generalizability of the psychoanalytic concept of the working alliance. *Psychotherapy: Theory, Research & Practice*, 16(3), 252.

Corrigan, P. W., & Phelan, S. M. (2004) Social support and recovery in people with serious mental illnesses. *Community Mental Health Journal*, 40(6), 513–23.

Hogarty, G. E., Anderson, C. M., Reiss, D. J., Kornblith, S. J., Greenwald, D. P., Javna, C. D., & Madonia, M. J. (1986) Family psychoeducation, social skills training, and maintenance chemotherapy in the aftercare treatment of schizophrenia. I. one-year effects of a controlled study on relapse and expressed emotion. *Archives of General Psychiatry*, 43(7), 633–42.

Jansen, J. E., Harder, S., Haahr, U. H., Lyse, H. G., Pedersen, M. B., Trauelsen, A. M., & Simonsen, E. (2015) The role of metacognitions in expressed emotion and distress: A study on caregivers of persons with first-episode psychosis. *Clinical Psychology & Psychotherapy*, 22(6), 525–32. doi:10.1002/cpp.1907 [doi]

Kane, J. M., Robinson, D. G., Schooler, N. R., et al. (2015) Comprehensive versus usual community care for first-episode psychosis: 2-year outcomes from the NIMH RAISE early treatment program. *American Journal of Psychiatry*, 173(4), 362–72.

Lowenstein, J. A., Butler, D. W., & Ashcroft, K. (2010) The efficacy of a cognitively orientated carers group in an early intervention in psychosis service—a pilot study. *Journal of Psychiatric and Mental Health Nursing*, 17(7), 628–35. doi:10.1111/j.1365-2850.2010.01564.x [doi]

Norcross, J. C., & Wampold, B. E. (2011) Evidence-based therapy relationships: Research conclusions and clinical practices. *Psychotherapy (Chicago, Ill.)*, 48(1), 98–102. doi:10.1037/a0022161 [doi]

Sadath, A., Muralidhar, D., Varambally, S., Gangadhar, B. N., & Jose, J. P. (2017) Do stress and support matter for caring? The role of perceived stress and social support on expressed emotion of carers of persons with first episode psychosis. *Asian Journal of Psychiatry*, 25, 163–8. doi:S1876-2018(15)30082-4 [pii]

Schoenbaum, M., Sutherland, J., Chappel, A., Azrin, S., Goldstein, A., Rupp, A., & Heinssen, R. (2017) Twelve-month health care use and mortality in commercially insured young people with incident psychosis in the United States. *Schizophrenia Bulletin*, 43(6), 1262–72.

Smith, J. V., & Birchwood, M. J. (1987) Specific and non-specific effects of educational intervention with families living with a schizophrenic relative. *The British Journal of Psychiatry : The Journal of Mental Science*, 150, 645–52.

Websites/Other Information

NAMI Programmes in the United States

The National Alliance on Mental Illness is the largest grassroots organisation dedicated to providing education, support and advocacy for individuals and families affected by mental illness. NAMI offers a wide range of free programmes run by trained facilitators who have lived experience with mental illness, either as a family member or as a peer (individuals living with mental illness). Some of the programmes are available in both Spanish and English.

One of NAMI's signature programmes is Family-to-Family, an intensive 12-week programme to facilitate a better understanding of mental illness and improve coping skills for families and friends of those with mental illness. Its topics include an understanding of mental illness and how it affects the brain, current science about medication and treatment, self-care for families, how to manage crises and problem-solve, how to communicate effectively with a loved one with mental illness and what resources are available to help families. This programme has been designated an evidence-based practice by the Substance Abuse and Mental Health Services Administration (SAMHSA).

Further Reading

Amador, X. F., & Johanson, A. L. (2000). *I am not sick, I don't need help!* New York, NY: Vida Press.

Lafond, V. (2002). *Grieving mental illness: A guide for patients and their caregivers*: Toronto, ON: University of Toronto Press.

Miklowitz, D. J. (2011). *The bipolar disorder survival guide: What you and your family need to know.* New York: Guilford Press.

Mueser, K. T., & Gingerich, S. (2006). *The complete family guide to schizophrenia: Helping your loved one get the most out of life.* New York: Guilford Press.

Torrey, E. F. (2013). *The indispensable guide to today's most misunderstood illness: Surviving schizophrenia: A manual for families, patients, and providers.* New York, NY: Harper Perennial.

Recommended Websites

Resources for Families/Carers in the United States

- www.nami.org/ – NAMI is a national organisation for family members and individuals with serious mental illness that provides support, education (including educational programmes for families) and advocacy.
- http://schizophrenia.com/ – This site describes itself as 'an Internet-based community' which provides a great deal of information from many perspectives, with a goal of supporting and educating family members, caregivers and individuals.
- www.nimh.nih.gov/health/topics/ schizophrenia/index.shtml – The National Institute of Mental Health (NIMH) is the lead federal agency for research on mental disorders, and its mission 'is to transform the understanding and treatment of mental illnesses through basic and clinical research, paving the way for prevention, recovery, and cure'.
- www.researchgate.net/ publication/235003455_Befriending_ Manual – This site has a link to a full copy of the *Befriending Manual*. Originally used as a control condition in research studies on treatment of psychosis, this manual offers useful tips that can be incorporated into everyday interactions between carers and service users to try to reduce distress and increase engagement.

- www.hearingvoicesusa.org/ – The Hearing Voices Network provides a support system for people who hear voices, including supporting local groups where the experiences of voices can be discussed without judgment or negative labelling, which can sometimes increase distress.
- www.intervoiceonline.org/ – Intervoice provides examples of different types of voices, coping strategies and information about Voice Hearing support groups.
- www.al-anon.alateen.org/ – Alanon was originally developed to provide social support to friends and families of individuals with a drug or alcohol misuse problem. However, many families that attend Alanon are also dealing with the combination of a severe mental disorder and a drug and alcohol problem so that Alanon groups are likely to be a quite useful source of support.
- www.treatingpsychosis.com/resources – This site provides a variety of informational and educational tools, including videos and websites inspiring hope for recovery. An excellent up-to-date resource for anyone affected by psychosis.
- http://navigateconsultants.org/ – This website describes a highly successful programme for people with early psychosis and their families and includes videos and other materials describing the treatment.
- www.ncbi.nlm.nih.gov/pubmed/ – This website provides no-cost access to research published in scholarly journals supported by the National Institutes of Health.

Index